PRAISE FOR
WHY IS MY KID DOING THAT?

"In 'Why is My Kid Doing That?', Cindy Utzinger identifies characteristics using scientific studies that enable her to offer adaptive learning strategies for those who may be "neurologically disorganized." (And who of us is not "neurologically disorganized" in some way and on some occasions?)

The conversational and personal tone Cindy uses invites readers who may not know the technical jargon to keep reading, and she offers numerous, practical alternatives for assisting children who are struggling to fit the mold. The examples of real children lend authenticity to all she says, and the scientific research offered is validated by her very own personal experience.

More and more children are facing neurological disorientation. Scientific data along with teacher and parental experience reflect that reality. Cindy's insight into this dilemma offers hope and promise to many."

- **EVELYN VEST-ARNOLD, ED.D.**

"This book literally came at a time when we were at a loss; concerned about our youngest's child's behavior and struggles with sensory related issues. What a lightbulb moment when Cindy so clearly demonstrates the tie between the two! This book put it so clearly into words to help us as parents understand how connected sensory and behavior are and most importantly, how to address it with care and knowledge. I'm so thankful for this book and can't wait to share with my fellow moms!"

- **BLAIR LAHAYE,** Parent and Former PR Executive

"Cindy did an amazing job writing a book that makes you feel like you are sitting and having a conversation with an Occupational Therapist. This book is packed with helpful information yet presented in a way that is practical and easy to understand. It is a valuable resource to help families to better understand the why behind their child's unique behaviors and I am excited to have this as a resource to share with the families that I work with."

- **LIANA M. HAMILTON, MS/OTR,** Occupational Therapist

"This is a wonderful book regarding sensory processing. It is very informative and would be great to have extra copies to give to family members and teachers. The only way people will learn more about children and how they relate differently due to sensory issues is by getting books like this in the hands of people who work with lots of kids. Cindy Utzinger has written this in easy to understand language that even someone who isn't familiar with sensory processing can understand. As both a teacher and a parent of a child with SPD, this book has helped me understand what my own child, and others, are going through and how to better reach them."

- **LEAH MCDOWELL,** 2nd Grade Teacher at Charlotte Mechlenburg School System

" As a parent resource consultant in the education field I love that Cindy Utzinger has brought this important information to parents. When your children are out of the box or as I say, have extra layers, it is important to understand every layer. Cindy has given you so much great information to help better understand each layer of your child. I wish I would have had this book to guide me when my girls were younger. Both of my girls have sensory processing and even as a professional with a child development degree I learned new things in Cindy's book. I will be recommending this book to all my clients! Thank you, Cindy for giving parents great information and guiding them so that their children can be their best! "

- **CASSIE BLAKELY,** Parent Resource Consultant

"Cindy Utzinger's book "Why Is My Kid Doing That?" has given me an abundance of knowledge and ideas for my role as a professional working with children with emotional and behavioral challenges as well as my role as a mother parenting a neuro-typically developing son. Her book has helped me to understand with much further clarity why some children may be acting out through emotions and behaviors and need more sensory interventions and not just mental health interventions and parenting work. She does an amazing job discussing the importance of building a sensory foundation and does an even better job at giving actual everyday ideas parents can utilize with their children (neurotypical or not) to help them with self-regulation and emotional and behavioral control. I will without a doubt recommend this to clients and mom friends!"

- **KARA L EWING, LCSW,** Mental Health Therapist

WHY IS MY KID DOING THAT?

WHY IS MY KID DOING THAT?

A Sensory Approach To Understanding Your Child's Behavior

CINDY UTZINGER, OTR/L

Why is My Kid Doing That?: A Sensory Approach to Understanding Your Child's Behavior
Copyright © 2019 by Cindy Utzinger
All Rights Reserved

This book is intended for general informational purposes only and is not meant to be used for, nor should it be used, to diagnose or treat any child. The advice and strategies contained in this book may not be suitable for all children and are intended to supplement, not replace, the advice of a trained medical professional. Please consult your healthcare provider before adopting any of the suggestions in this book, as well as, for any questions that you may have regarding your child's medical situation. Readers of this book are responsible for their own safety and the safety of the children in their care. The author and publisher of this book disclaim any liability arising directly or indirectly from the use of this book.

All rights reserved. No part of this publication may be reproduced, distributed, or transmitted in any form or by any means, including photocopying, recording, or other electronic or mechanical methods, without the prior written permission of the publisher or author, except in the case of brief quotations embodied in critical reviews and certain other noncommercial uses permitted by copyright law. For permission requests, email the publisher or author at info@cindyutzinger.com.

Copy editor © Andrea C. Jasmin
www.acjasminproofreading.com
Front and back cover design © Melissa Clampitt
www.melissaclampittdesigns.com
Interior book design © Melissa Clampitt
www.melissaclampittdesigns.com
Front cover photo by © Sunny studio

Back cover photo © Heather Rasmussen
www.heatherrasmussenphotography.com

To contact the publisher, visit
www.cindyutzinger.com
To contact author, visit
www.cindyutzinger.com

ISBN 13: 978-1698468693

Some names have been changed to protect the privacy of the individuals involved.

Printed in the United States of America

DEDICATION

To my favorite kids, Britton and Lauren. Thank you for teaching me the capacity of a mama's heart to love. You two brighten the world and I cherish the privilege of being able to ask myself "Why is my kid doing that?".

TABLE OF CONTENTS

DEDICATION vii
ACKNOWLEDGMENTS xi
FOREWORD xiii
INTRODUCTION xv

SECTION 1: CHILD DEVELOPMENT 101 0
    CHAPTER 1: SENSORY FOUNDATION 1
    CHAPTER 2: THE SENSORY FOUNDATION 101 3
    CHAPTER 3: WHERE THE QUIRKS LURK 12
    CHAPTER 4: THE FEEDBACK LOOP 15
    CHAPTER 5: TURN ON THE AUTOPILOT 17
    CHAPTER 6: SENSORY INTEGRATION...WHAT? 20

SECTION 2: LET'S GET TO THE WHY 24
    CHAPTER 7: IT'S A DIFFERENT WORLD WE LIVE IN 25
    CHAPTER 8: THE SENSORY UMBRELLA 31
    CHAPTER 9: THE SENSORY CUPS 34
    CHAPTER 10: OPTIMUM LEVEL OF AROUSAL AND SELF-REGULATION 37
    CHAPTER 11: THE IMMATURE SENSORY SYSTEM 41
    CHAPTER 12: THE PROPRIOCEPTIVE (pro-pri-o-cep-tive) SYSTEM 46
    CHAPTER 13: THE VESTIBULAR (vest-tib-u-lar) SYSTEM 52
    CHAPTER 14: THE TACTILE (tac-tile) SYSTEM 59
    CHAPTER 15: SENSORY PROCESSING DISORDER 66
    CHAPTER 16: ADD/ADHD AND THE SENSORY SYSTEM 77
    CHAPTER 17: AUTISM SPECTRUM DISORDER AND THE SENSORY SYSTEM 85
    CHAPTER 18: FEARS, ANXIETY, MELTDOWNS, OR DIFFICULTY WITH TRANSITIONS 91

TABLE OF CONTENTS

CHAPTER 19: GROWTH SPURTS = REGRESSION 95

SECTION 3: THERE IS HOPE - HOW TO HELP YOUR CHILDREN 98

CHAPTER 20: THE BRAIN CAN CHANGE 99

CHAPTER 21: A FEW SENSORY QUESTIONS TO ASK YOURSELF 102

CHAPTER 22: WORKING SENSORY INPUT IN TO AN ALREADY BUSY DAY 104

CHAPTER 23: PROPRIOCEPTIVE ACTIVITIES 113

CHAPTER 24: VESTIBULAR ACTIVITIES 115

CHAPTER 25: TACTILE ACTIVITIES 117

CHAPTER 26: STRATEGIES TO USE WITH CHILDREN WHO ARE SENSORY UNDER-SENSITIVE 120

CHAPTER 27: STRATEGIES TO USE WITH CHILDREN WHO ARE SENSORY OVER- SENSITIVE 123

CHAPTER 28: ADD/ADHD ACTIVITIES 127

CHAPTER 29: SELF-REGULATION/CALMING ACTIVITIES 129

CONCLUSION 134

APPENDIX A: SENSORY CHECKLIST 136

BIBLIOGRAPHY 145

ACKNOWLEDGMENTS

This is by far the most difficult section of the book to write because there are so many people who have been by my side to support and encourage me to help me get to this point. To each one of you who lent me your ear (You know who you are!), thank you!

To my amazing family, thank you for all your support and encouragement. Britton and Lauren, there's nothing I love more in this world than being your mom and watching you grow into amazing young people. Thank you for sharing me with so many other children and for your patience with me as I wrote this book. I love you guys more than words can say.

To my Eric. Thank you, thank you, thank you for your support, understanding, sacrifice, and patience throughout the process of writing this book (and over the last 18 years in general). Thank you for letting me do this even when it seemed like a crazy dream. This book would have never happened if you wouldn't have put up with the sound of me typing in bed every night as you tried to fall asleep. I love you!

To my mom and dad. Thank you for giving me the tools I needed to succeed in life, and more than anything, for your love and support. Dad, this book would still be sitting in my "saved" folder if it wasn't for your pushing me.

To my beautiful sisters Marcie DeMore and Jodi Jones. Thank you for putting up with me and listening. A special thanks, Marcie, for helping me with edits and making decisions when my thoughts were swirling over choices while putting together the finishing touches.

To my editor and coach, Andrea Jasmin. Your encouragement and cheerleading gave me confidence just at the right times. You took me from fear to peace and helped me learn to think big. It's no coincidence our sons ended up on the same soccer team!

To my cover designer and interior book designer, Melissa Clampitt. Thank you for your amazing amount of patience in trying to figure me out and get inside of my head to see my vision and get the design just right.

To the person who sparked this fire, Tim Vest. I thought you were crazy when you said I should write a book. I may or may not have cursed you a few times throughout this process, but, without you, I never would have thought that I had it in me. So, my apologies for cursing you and thank you for the push and believing

ACKNOWLEDGMENTS

I could do this. Thank you, also, for volunteering your mom Dr. Evelyn Vest- Arnold to help me. I appreciate all your time and advice, Evelyn, in the early days of this venture. You were instrumental in getting this book off the ground.

To my "Homies." I count my blessings for you ladies every day. Thank you Karen White, Ashley Williams, Amanda Logan, Elizabeth Austin, and Michelle Gervasini for helping me to stay strong as a wife and mother through your support and friendship.

To my colleagues. Liane Hamilton, Cari Fresoli, Gail Kalstek, and April Lane. Thank you for helping me to learn and grow as an Occupational Therapist and being the most amazing group of ladies to work with that a girl could ever ask for.

To everyone else at Lake Norman Children's Therapy. I love each one of you ladies and count it a real privilege to get to collaborate with you. I can't think of a better place to work or a more amazing group of ladies to work with. Jenny Plummer, Keri Poe, Susan McCoy, Angie Munch, Taylor Miller, Heather Wesseler, Julie Kouzel, Liza Gosnell, and Cheryl Nowak you are a bright light to my workday.

To my friends. Kate Kester, thanks for the long walks and talks that keep me lifted up yet grounded at the same time. Tara Setzer, thank you for listening to all my swirling thoughts and helping me make decisions. Jeanie Mason, thank you for your prayers, guidance, and support. Without it, I think I'd still be spinning in circles. Lee Steinour, thanks for bringing me in to the twenty-first century by teaching me how to use social media and talking me through book designs. Cara and John Stanford, thanks for your support, encouragement, and teaching me to think with a business mind.

To my amazing endorsers. Blair Lahaye, Cassie Blakely, Liane Hamilton, Kara Ewing, Leah McDowell, Dr. Evelyn Vest-Arnold, Gemma Medina, Marlynn Love, and Jennifer Frazier, thank you for your time, support, and honesty. You have helped give this book (and me) wings to fly.

To my technology guys. Chuck Austin and Tim Morin, thank you for being so gracious in building cindyutzinger.com. Your patience with me and generosity with your time mean more to me than words could express. You two added years back on to my life.

To all the uniquely gifted children and their parents whom I have had the opportunity to work with over the years. Thank you for trusting me and for allowing me to grow in knowledge through the experience of working with you. You all have a special place in my heart and are what made this book happen.

To you, the reader. Thank you for letting me in to your home or classroom and trusting me. Together, we can do this!

FOREWORD

"Why is My Kid Doing That?" is a question that is an inevitable part of parenting a child. One that we have become accustomed to not getting the answer to and chalking it up to having a "high-energy," "quirky," or "difficult" child. But what if you could have an understanding . . . an awareness . . . tools to arm yourself with during those frustrating moments? That's what Cindy Utzinger has offered in this book. It turns out that we all have what she explains as a sensory foundation and she breaks down why various behaviors take place, how to understand them, and tools to provide an outlet for them.

We all have those things that get us super excited and fired up! Things that we could talk about for hours because we are so passionate about it. We've learned it, we've mastered it, we've researched it constantly, and so at any chance, we share what we know and teach it. Sensory awareness is Cindy's "thing." In Cindy's case sometimes that teaching looks formal, such as working with clients in a clinic setting or advising teachers on the occupational therapy needs of a student, and sometimes that teaching looks informal like sharing advice with a struggling mom friend.

I had the privilege of working with Cindy as her editor for this book. Getting to be a witness to someone living their truth by sharing their gifts and knowledge it is a beautiful thing. It takes vulnerability to write a book. It feels natural to share with a friend or do the work we've been trained to do, but a book? That's a different story. Self-doubt is alive and well in all of us and so the reason for embarking on the process of writing a book has to be bigger than you. You have to feel compelled to do it because you feel deep down that you can help people with the knowledge you have. Cindy was clearly called to write this book. In the pages of this book you'll see firsthand the way that she has educated herself, pulled from her experience as an Occupational Therapist for the past 21 years, and shared examples from parenting her own two children. She's presented it all in a manner that feels authentic, intimate, and informative. She offers answers and hope. We all get to benefit from Cindy stepping out of her comfort zone with this gift to gain a better understanding of the sensory world.

When you share your skills with a community, as she has done, it's not just a book that is birthed at the end, it's service work; it's an offering. It's serving your community though recognizing your obligation to share what you've been blessed

FOREWORD

to be an expert on in a way that only you can. Cindy's approach to educating parents and educators through this book has her unique touch all over it. She approaches your hard to understand questions with empathy and delicate hands through her explanations that—while sometimes technical to make sure you understand the science behind everything—are also relatable and will leave you well informed and inspired.

I am a mother of two children and one of my children, as a toddler, needed daily playground time, struggled through transition times like leaving pre-school at the end of the day, acted impulsively, but could also focus to play a game of chess. As a new mother I would have given anything for a book that could have acted as a guide and helped me to understand that not only was I not alone but that all children have sensory needs! (Even those without an official diagnosis.) Every parent reading this will think "That's my child!" at least once. And as a tool for educators it will give you perspective, understanding, and concrete suggestions to better support your classroom.

Prepare to have many "ah-ha" moments as you dive into "Why is My Kid Doing That?" and learn the "Why?" from a woman that so graciously has taken her years of experience and expertise and broken down all things sensory. It turns out that the children in our lives have real reasons behind what they do and it's actually not just to drive us mad! Enjoy!

ANDREA C. JASMIN, Copy Editor, Proofreader & Book Coach

INTRODUCTION

If there is one phrase from my childhood that my dad used to say over and over, it's this: "There is no handbook for parenting, Cindy. Your mom and I are just learning as we go." There are actually a lot of things my dad used to say that make a lot more sense now that I am a parent, but that one sure seems to stand out. If only there were a step by step handbook for raising kids; how much easier would life be? Well, there isn't a handbook or recipe that is right for each child, so that leaves us all just doing the best we can and crossing our fingers that our children turn out OK.

While this book is by no means a parenting or child rearing handbook, my purpose in writing it is to help make it at least a little bit easier on you. In order to do this, I want to help you to gain more understanding of WHY your children may act or behave in certain ways and then help you know WHAT you can do about it. Let me begin by telling you a little bit about myself and why I felt compelled to write this book.

I am a wife and mother of two children. My children are both what you would consider "typically developing" children. However, they are children, and we know there is no such thing as a perfect child (Sorry, Kids!). On a daily basis, I see firsthand what can happen to children when they are, what I like to call, "neurologically disorganized." By this I mean those times when they are in the heat of a tantrum, when they can't focus, or when they just can't seem to control their own behaviors or emotions. These occurrences may take place when they are getting ready for school, doing school work, during a meal, riding in the car, playing with friends, and they may happen as many as a million other times during the day (or so it sometimes seems). As a mom I want to be able to fix whatever problem is going on in my children's lives, but, unfortunately, I can't. Because of the knowledge that I have through my studies and experience as an OT, I may not always be able to fix things for my children, but I have a pretty good bag of tricks of things to do to help them. It is now my privilege to be able to share this with you.

That leads me, then, into explaining to you why I wrote this book. As an Occupational Therapist, I work with children in their homes, in an outpatient clinic, and in schools who have Sensory Processing Disorder, ADD/ADHD, developmental delays, or autism spectrum disorder. In doing so, I can see the

INTRODUCTION

frustration and sense parents being overwhelmed and not knowing what to do to help their children when they are struggling with motor skills, behaviors, academic skills, peer relations, etc. I hear the frustration in teachers' voices when they have a child in their classroom who doesn't quite fit the mold and they don't know what to do to help them.

My first goal in writing this book is to help you as parents, caregivers, and educators to take a deep breath and feel a sense of hope. I want you to understand *why* your children are doing what they are doing. I want you to understand what is often the root cause for a behavior or deficit they are showing in the classroom. I hear so many parents say "If I would have known." They will express that they knew their children had some "quirks", "problems", or "differences" but didn't know exactly what was going on or what to do about it. That leads me to my second goal which is to help you to know *what* to do to help them. I want you to feel empowered. When you start seeing a pattern of behavior that is undesirable, when your child's teacher raises concerns about performance or behavior in the classroom, or when you see your child is lagging behind peers with motor skills, for you to say "I've got this" instead of a sense of feeling overwhelmed and not knowing where to turn to help.

This book is for any parent, caregiver, or teacher who has or works with "typically developing" children or who has or works with those who have been given a diagnosis. This book is for people with "typically developing" children who want to help give their children the boost that every kid needs, to ensure that they have a strong foundation (sensory foundation) for building skills. This book is also for parents, caregivers, or teachers who realize that their own children or one they know or supervise has worrisome quirks, and due to their responsibility to these children, they want to make sense of it. Last, but not least, this book is for parents, caregivers, or teachers who have children or work with children who have been given a diagnosis of SPD, developmental delay, ADD/ADHD, or children with autism spectrum disorder to use in conjunction with the other therapies and services they are receiving. I have heard many parents complain that they have this nice long evaluation that was written up by their children's therapist but that, unfortunately, it doesn't make any sense to them. This is to help you make heads and tails of what is going on with those children, what those big words on that evaluation mean, and empower you to help them on a day-to-day basis.

LET'S GET STARTED!

SECTION 1:

CHILD DEVELOPMENT 101

CHAPTER 1

SENSORY FOUNDATION

You Can Huff And Puff But You Can't Blow This House Down

"Why is my kid doing that?" That is the million dollar question! To help you gain answers, I would like to share with you an overview of how the sensory system works and how children learn. To do so, I like to use building blocks as a visual. I like to call them the building blocks of learning. The reason for this is that the way children learn and develop skills can be compared to building a tower of blocks; without a good foundation, the blocks will topple over. For a moment, I want to also use the example of constructing a building to learning and developing skills as we all know how important a good foundation is to the structure of a building.

When a building is constructed, tremendous time, attention, and materials are put into forming the foundation of the building (the part we often don't even see). The land has to be graded so it is level, pilings have to be strategically placed to support the structure, a cement foundation has to be laid, etc., all so the building will be strong, have a good solid base, and not collapse with time as the ground shifts or when a big storm hits. This important step can, and should, take a lot of time and planning.

A few years ago, there was a new elementary school being built right outside of our neighborhood. We drove by it several times every day and my kids were so excited watching it being built knowing they would both go there one day. The question I would hear every time we drove by was "When will they be done building it?" You see, the construction crews had been out there working on it for four months and there was still not much to look at other than dirt, cinder blocks, and a bunch of diggers, bulldozers, and other trucks that I have no idea what their purpose is. To the naked eye, it did not appear that they were moving along very quickly. However, even with my minimal knowledge of construction, I knew that what they were doing was one of the most important aspects of building that school. They were working on laying a very strong foundation on which to erect it. At least I hope. If not, we will be in big trouble later!

Think about the *Three Little Pigs*. Which house withstood the big bad wolf? The house that was built of strong materials and had a sturdy foundation! All the big bad wolf had to do was "huff and puff" and he was able to blow the two houses down that weren't built with sturdy materials.

Once a good solid foundation is laid, a big, beautiful structure can be built. As onlookers or spectators, we generally don't give the foundation a second thought. We just enjoy the beautiful skyscraper (or in the case of me and my children, the new school) being built. We pay attention to the part we see, not the foundation which we don't see.

That is how we can think of learning. The foundation is what is so important and is where initial learning actually occurs. It is basic to all other learning, yet we often don't pay much attention to it. Where we tend to focus our attention is on the top of the building, the part with all of the pretty windows and neat designs. With our children, the top of the building is what we see children do, their performance, and behaviors. We see their behaviors, how they control their emotions, how they perform in school or on the ball field, and while playing with friends. We see their ability or inability to sit and focus, learn a new task, hold a pencil, catch a ball, ride a bike, etc. What we need to realize is that these skills were all built (or formed) from their foundation. When there is a faulty learning foundation, the part we see (their performance) often struggles to hold up, or be, where it needs to be. Children will always learn and develop; however, without the proper foundation, they will learn and develop faulty patterns. The key is; however, not necessarily to try to fix their performance, but to go back and look at the foundation and make the necessary changes there.

Go back to our building for a minute. If it were starting to lean, we wouldn't put stakes in place to try to prop it up. Instead, we would go back and look at the foundation, realizing that the problem is occurring there. Perhaps the ground wasn't level or the pilings weren't put in place correctly. If we just tried to prop the building up, we would be putting a Band-Aid on the problem which would just be a temporary fix. Similarly, in learning we need to go straight to the foundation and give it the necessary boost that it needs.

CHAPTER 2

THE SENSORY FOUNDATION 101

My goal when writing this book was to keep it very simple and easy to understand. Please bare with me but I have to get a little technical here so you have all the information you need to understand the "Why?".

Since we know that the foundation for learning is so important, I want to spend some time explaining what makes up the foundation. The blocks that form the base of the building blocks of learning, or the foundation of our pyramid, are where learning occurs. The blocks at the top of the building blocks are made up of their performance, what we see our children do.

DNA Make-Up – The first block that lays the foundation of the building blocks is our DNA. DNA contains all of the genetic instructions used in the development and functioning of living organisms. Our hair color, eye color, shape of our nose, height, and so on, are determined by our DNA. Our DNA is obviously out of our control as it is what we are born with. In the "nature vs nurture" argument, DNA is our "nature." I will talk more about ADD, ADHD, and the autism spectrum in later chapters but want to mention here that researchers feel DNA may likely play a role in both.

Reflex Maturation (Integration) – The next block in the foundation is the maturation of our primitive reflexes. Primitive reflexes are involuntary movement patterns seen during infancy which equip infants with innate survival skills. These reflexes appear in infancy and then mature, or integrate in to *voluntary movement patterns* that are consciously controlled. This happens as the infant moves and develops new skills and becomes more organized no longer needing the reflexes. An example of this is the sucking reflex. The sucking reflex helps newborns to fulfill their basic need of receiving nutrition as they suck in response to something being placed in their mouths or to being touched around their mouths. Around 2-3 months of age this reflex will mature, or integrate, as the infant begins to suck out of conscious effort as opposed to its being a reflexive action.

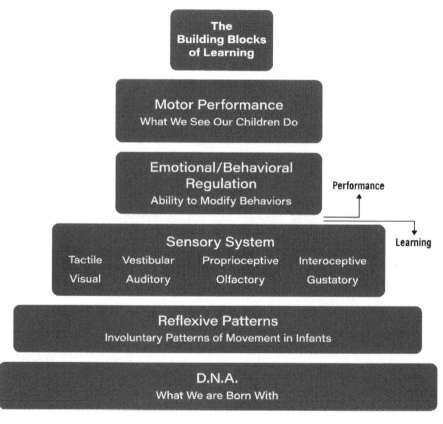

The Learning Triangle adapted from Strauss 1985; Oden 2002

While there are some reflexes that are seen even in adulthood (for example, yawning, blinking, and coughing), there are reflexes, such as the ones that help infants learn to suck, grasp, roll over, crawl, and move against gravity, that need to integrate in to voluntary movements. Once infants have opportunities to move around and interact with the world around them, they no longer need these reflexes and the voluntary movements they have learned become part of their repertoire.

When these reflexes mature into voluntary movements that they now consciously control, this becomes a foundation for movement and stability, a foundation off which all movements occur. When this has not successfully occurred, you may see such things as postural weakness, difficulty with fine motor and gross motor coordination, difficulty sitting upright in a chair, or clumsiness. Other signs of faulty reflex maturation can be difficulty with skills such as handwriting or catching a ball.

Children will continue to grow and develop even when their reflexes have not fully matured; however, they will develop faulty patterns for doing things. An example of this is children who struggle to sit up straight in their seat at their desk. Slumping over, propping their head on their hand or arm, or slouching in their seat with their legs wrapped around the legs of the chair are signs we should pay attention to. If you remember back to when your children were infants, they were more than likely either curled up like a ball when they were on their stomachs or lying stretched out when they were on their backs. Believe it or not, reflexes are responsible for that. When the reflexes (the labyrinthine reflexes) that cause babies to lie in those positions have not successfully matured from involuntary movements to voluntary, maintaining good trunk control to sit up straight in a chair is very difficult.

Sensory System – The remainder of the foundation is made up of the sensory system which is composed of the eight senses. There are the basic senses with which we are all familiar: sight, smell, sound, taste, and touch. These senses receive and respond to information children receive externally from their environment. There are also senses with which we are less familiar, senses that respond to information gathered from *within* children's bodies. In the *Out Of Sync Child* (Kranowitz 2006), Kranowitz refers to them as our "near senses" since we cannot observe them and they happen without conscious thought.

The "near senses" include the proprioceptive, vestibular, tactile, and interoceptive systems, and I will spend a little more time explaining these because the majority of us are unfamiliar with them. The "near senses," and in particular the proprioceptive, vestibular, and tactile systems, form a very large portion of the sensory foundation and must come together to form our kinesthetic awareness, including our body awareness, our concept of what our body is doing in space, and to give us a concept of personal space. When these systems don't come together successfully, you will see children start to fall apart, often leading to behavior problems.

The **"near senses"** include the following sensory systems:

Proprioceptive (pro-preo-sep-tiv) System – This is our "position" sense as it processes the information gathered through our muscles, ligaments, and joints to tell us the position of our body. This sense helps us to understand our movements through the information our brain receives when our muscles or joints are stressed or "loaded." Proprioceptive information is gathered through the stretching or contracting of our muscles or bending, straightening, pulling, and compressing our joints.

Our proprioceptive sense lets us know that our elbow is bent vs. straight even when we can't see it. It helps us to put one foot in front of the other in order to walk without having to look at our feet. Two good examples of activities in which we receive proprioceptive input, are jumping and running. Think of all of the proprioceptive input our brains receive during these activities as the muscles and ligaments in our legs and trunk contract and as our joints are compressed as our feet strike or hit the ground. When we crab walk or do push-ups, we get great proprioceptive input through our arms due to the amount of weight we bear through them during these activities. The resistance our muscles receive when carrying heavy objects provides proprioceptive input, as well as, when deep pressure is applied to our muscles during a deep massage or big bear hug.

An intact proprioceptive system and an understanding of where our body parts are in relation to our surroundings, make it possible for us to carry out gross motor and fine motor skills (examples include kicking a ball, riding a bike, writing legibly, using a fork to feed ourselves, or using scissors to cut). Most of our proprioceptive sense occurs unconsciously; therefore, allowing us to perform a motor task without having to watch our limbs to know what they are doing. Think about hitting a baseball—people need to be able to know what their arms are doing while swinging a bat without watching them so they can keep their eye on the ball. If you had to watch your arms swing the bat instead of watching the ball, it would make baseball a much more dangerous sport!

Proprioception also gives us the ability to "grade" and time our movements. That means it helps us know if we need to use more or less force, move our limbs faster or slower, use bigger or smaller movements, etc. Again, think of the baseball example—while watching the ball, and not the bat or your arms, you have to determine if you need to swing the bat higher or lower, how forcefully to swing the bat, and when to swing the bat. A lot goes on unconsciously to hit that baseball (or perform most motor skills for that matter)—a lot that we take for granted when we don't have to consciously think about it. Another example of "grading" our movements is judging how much pressure to use when holding a Styrofoam cup. You have to squeeze it tightly enough not to drop it, but if you squeeze it too hard, you will crush it.

I want to also mention here that proprioceptive input can be calming and neurologically organizing. By neurologically organizing, I mean that it helps to get our brains prepped and ready to go, or learn. For me it is running or exercise in general. My brain gets prepped and is ready to focus after I exercise or go for a nice long run. Knowing that proprioceptive input is calming and neurologically organizing is going to be important to help you understand more as you read on. For now, just store in the back of your mind the idea that when you see that your children need calming or assistance with self-organization, you can give them opportunities to receive proprioceptive input.

Vestibular System – The vestibular system gathers information through a mechanism in the inner ear called the "vestibule." It is anatomically joined to the cochlear system (which is dedicated to hearing), and it tells us where our head is in relation to gravity by processing changes in head position. Both movement of our heads and gravity stimulate the vestibular receptors. This means that it is not just movement that stimulates the receptors but that simply the act of holding our heads up against gravity gives the vestibular system input.

This system is so important because it helps us to develop a sense of what our bodies are doing in relationship to the rest of the world and to comprehend that. The vestibular system also provides the foundation for many other functions and helps prepare our nervous system for input received from our other senses such as our eyes, ears, muscles, and joints. This system plays a role in motivation and attention and is what Jean Ayres (1979) called the "unifying system." Visual, auditory, proprioceptive, and tactile messages all get tied back to the vestibular system to help us make sense of it. For example, when we hear a noise, we have to know where we are in relation to that noise to determine where it came from. When we see a car go by, we have to know how fast we are moving to realize whether the car that passed us was going fast or slow. Trott, Laurel, and Windeck (1993) state that "Vestibular input tells us whether or not we are moving, how quickly we are moving and in what direction we are moving. It provides us with that sense of safety that can only come from knowing that one's feet are planted firmly on the ground." In addition to letting us know how we are moving, this system allows us to know whether an object is moving, or motionless, in relationship to our bodies.

Let me give you an example of what it can be like when there is a kink in this system. The other day I had my car washed in one of those car washes at a gas station where the car is stationary, but the large rotating brushes that wash the car and the entire mechanism they are attached to move forward and backward as it cleans the car. Oh my goodness! I am watching this thing and the next thing you know I have a headache and am dizzy. So you know I had to start analyzing this situation! I realized that my visual system and vestibular system were at war. It looked visually like the car was moving, but it wasn't. So my eyes were telling my brain that I was moving, but my vestibular system was not registering that I was moving (because I wasn't). The visual information I was receiving was getting tied back to the vestibular information I was receiving, but somehow they were at a tug-o-war and I was paying the price for it as I experienced a headache and nausea because of it.

Another important role of the vestibular system is in influencing our muscle tone since it tells muscles how much they need to contract to counteract gravity. Muscle tone is the normal level of muscle *tension* and is very different from muscle *strength*. When children's muscle tone is affected by their vestibular system, it can often make them appear "floppy" or make their arms and legs appear to be weak (Again, remember it is not weakness; however, it is muscle tone that is playing a role here.) I will talk more about this in Chapter 13 when I discuss problems with the vestibular system.

The vestibular system enables the two sides of our bodies to communicate to the brain in a way that allows us to use both our left and right sides together in a coordinated manner (*bilateral coordination*). Think about all of the activities that your children do that require them to use both arms together in a coordinated manner. Holding a shovel in one hand and a bucket in the other to scoop sand into the bucket, using one hand to hold the paper steady while using the other hand to write or cut with scissors, holding their lunch or school bag in one hand while using the other to unzip it, tying shoes, catching and throwing are all examples of activities that require bilateral coordination.

Before I explain the next "near sense," I want to pause here and make an important point about the vestibular and proprioceptive systems. Together, these systems allow our children to know what their bodies are doing in space, as well as where their bodies are in space. An understanding of "where I am" in space involves posture, timing, rhythm, balance, and understanding the qualities of their movements. This understanding forms the foundation for all other skills and learning including reading, math, spelling, fine motor and gross motor coordination, communication skills, and any other skill you can think of.

A knowledge of "where I am" gives children a greater sense of confidence. I'm sure you can imagine how challenging it is for a child to navigate through their day and through life without a clear understanding of this. When a child is not clear on where their body is in relation to the world around them, it can throw even the simplest of tasks off. How loud/quiet do I talk? How do I make my body climb that equipment? How do I sit in that chair without falling out? How do I step over that? How hard do I throw that ball to that person standing over there? How do I keep my balance to ride my bike? How do I use my body to play with that child without hurting them?

Tactile System – The next "near sense" is the tactile sense. This is our touch system and is our largest sensory system since it is gathered through our largest organ (our skin). Our tactile system is important from the moment we are born because it helps babies bond with and feel secure with the people who love them. This system processes information regarding touch, temperature, texture, vibration, and pain.

The tactile system has two subsystems which are important to understand because they play an important role in behavior. The first is the **discriminative system**. This system gives us the information regarding the qualities of a tactile stimulus such as whether it is hot or cold, soft or hard, giving us deep or light pressure, bumpy or smooth, painful or pleasant, etc. When this system is intact, we can hold an object in our hand and, without seeing it, be able to figure out what it is by feeling the qualities of it. Someone could place a quarter in your hand and, without seeing it, you could figure out that it is a quarter. You could feel that it is cold like metal, round, has ridges around the outside, know it is larger than a dime, etc. This system plays an important role in the development of fine motor skills. You have to understand the tactile information you are receiving in order to properly utilize a pencil for handwriting, manipulate a fork or spoon during mealtime, manipulate a button or zipper when dressing, etc.

The second subsystem is the **protective system**. The protective system is very powerful as it warns us of danger. It is connected to our autonomic nervous system (or our involuntary nervous system) and puts us on high alert or makes us respond quickly and emotionally to a stimulus that we perceive as being harmful. This is the system that makes us jump back quickly if we touch a hot stove or makes our hearts start pounding, makes us start to sweat, and then quickly swat at our leg when we feel an insect crawling on it. The reason we respond this way without even having to think about it is that our autonomic nervous system kicks us in to "fight, flight, or fright" mode when we perceive a stimulus to be harmful or noxious. This leads us to move quickly in an attempt to avoid a potentially dangerous situation.

Interoceptive System – The last of the "near senses" in our interoceptive sense. This system provides us with sensations from internal sensors near our organs including our heart, stomach, bowel, and bladder. It tells us how we feel inside as it gives us information regarding our heart rate, hunger, thirst, digestion, state of arousal, mood, etc. Because this system involves the bowel and bladder, it is also important for potty training and feeling when our bladder is full and recognizing the urge to urinate or when the intestine is active and we need to have a bowel movement.

The **external senses** include the following:

Visual System – This system involves the information brought in from the eyes. Important in determining where we are in space, it works with the vestibular, proprioceptive, and tactile systems. Together they allow us to make sense of the world around us and perform motor actions related to what we see (ex. hitting a baseball).

Auditory System – This system involves the information gathered through our ears. Processing of auditory information includes the ability to separate sounds heard in one ear from the other and allows us to discern sounds (such as distinguishing mom talking while the TV is turned on, the sound of the teacher's voice from background noise in the classroom, or the sound that "b" makes vs. "v").

Olfactory System – This system refers to our sense of smell and can affect our emotions, allow us to know if we are in danger, and help us enjoy what we are eating. This is what allows us to identify a meal without seeing it, panic when we smell smoke, or smell a perfume and remember somebody else that would wear that same perfume (whether it conjures up good memories or bad).

Gustatory System – This is our taste sense. The five types of gustatory receptors are sweet, sour, spicy, bitter, or savory. The gustatory sense allows us to distinguish between safe and harmful foods or pleasurable and non-pleasurable foods. For example, bitter and sour foods are usually unpleasant to us while sweet, salty, and savory foods give us a pleasurable sensation.

There is room for error in each one of these senses as children may be over or under-sensitive (or over or under responsive) to the information gathered from each. I will discuss this more in chapters to come and specifically focus on the proprioceptive, vestibular, and tactile senses. I want you to tuck away this basic understanding of the sensory systems to help you make sense of the following chapters.

CHAPTER 3

WHERE THE QUIRKS LURK

Now that we have identified and discussed the foundational layers of the building blocks, the layers where learning occurs, let's now identify and discuss the layers or blocks that are more visible to us. We can't see what is going on beneath the surface when it comes to our childrens' sensory system but what we do see is how they act behaviorally and emotionally and how well they are able to perform at the tasks in front of them. These are the layers of the building blocks where we see those quirky behaviors start to poke their ugly heads out.

Emotional/behavioral regulation – This describes children's ability to self-regulate or modify their behaviors and emotions. Children need to be able to self-regulate in response to their surroundings and circumstances and any changes that may take place to them. Self-regulation takes place from moment to moment. This may include the ability to tolerate transitions, develop appropriate attention span, control impulses, have self-control, sit still in class, calm oneself when overstimulated or upset, and the ability to form and maintain peer relationships. Children who can self-regulate will avoid throwing tantrums, instead being able to remain calm despite overstimulating circumstances, things not going their way, or changes to their routine.

The ability to self-regulate can help build children's self-esteem and the reverse is also true. Children who lack self-regulation skills will often suffer a breakdown in self-esteem.

Motor responses, patterns, and skills – Motor performance is the top layer of our building blocks and is comprised of motor responses, motor patterns, and motor skills. These terms can be described in the following way:

- **Motor response**: A voluntary movement in response to a stimulus (information the brain receives from our senses). To break this down into layman's terms, let's think of a baby learning to walk. His first motor response is to voluntarily lift his foot off the ground to take a step towards reaching that much desired toy he just laid eyes on.

- **Motor pattern**: A particular sequence of muscle movements that is directed at accomplishing a goal. A motor pattern is more refined than a motor response. This takes place when we make a motor response (the baby trying to take a step) then make adjustments (or recalculations) to that response based on the feedback our senses give us regarding the outcome of that response. Whoops! The baby fell. Next time he will recalculate his balance, how high to lift his foot, or his speed in moving based on the feedback that he received from his last effort. "Hmmm. I might need to pick my foot up higher next time, not lean so far forward, and bring my feet a little closer together. Let me try that and see if I can do this without falling!"
- **Motor skill**: This is a learned sequence of movements that combine to produce a smooth, efficient action in order to master a task. This is a highly refined pattern of movement that is based off of continuous incoming information, adjustments made, and experience. Look at baby go! All of that falling paid off. He can now walk without holding on to anything and without falling. He has developed a new motor skill. He practiced over and over again for months, taking a few more steps each time, and making re-calculations each time in order to further his distance—learning how to put one foot in front of the other, learning how high to lift that foot each time, and learning to control his trunk for balance. Soon, he'll put this process back in action to learn to run!

Everything we do requires this sequence—running, jumping, riding a bike, kicking or hitting a ball, sitting in a chair, writing, using utensils to eat, our speech, the list goes on. These activities all require the process of making a motor response, making adjustments to turn it in to a motor pattern, then refining it further to turn it in to a motor skill from which we will then build and refine even more.

The process of developing motor skills also requires **motor planning**. This means children have to come up with the idea of what they want to do, formulate a plan, organize the steps involved in getting it done, and then execute the motor skills involved. Motor planning is the ability to conceive the idea of what to do ("I want to walk."), planning what to do ("I need to lift my feet off the ground one at a time and keep my balance."), and then perform the movement or task ("Look at me. I'm walking.").

Proper and effective motor planning and developing efficient motor skills do not happen automatically. They are learned. And where does learning occur? I'll give you a hint—at the foundation of the building blocks. That's right. Learning occurs at our foundation and through the sensory input we get from movement and experiences gained from exploring our environment. Sure, we can all form motor skills, but if the foundation isn't laid or isn't strong enough, these motor skills will be based on, what Athena Oden (2006) calls, faulty and adaptive patterns. We will be able to perform but, chances are, not as well as we would like to or as well as what is expected of us.

> Proper and effective motor planning and developing efficient motor skills do not happen automatically. THEY ARE LEARNED.

CHAPTER 4

THE FEEDBACK LOOP

The foundation of the building blocks (DNA make-up, reflex maturation, and the eight senses) is the intangible layer that lays the foundation for children's motor skills and their ability to regulate their emotions and behaviors. What I can't stress enough, is that basic learning occurs at the foundation of the building blocks and performance occurs at the top part. However, they are a constant feedback loop. By this I mean that children's foundation influences their performance and the feedback that they receive about their performance (through others reactions, their outcomes, their senses, etc.) helps to further build their foundation.

It is also important to point out that the building blocks are not meant to represent a hierarchy where each system has to be fully developed in order for the next system to develop. Instead, the building blocks are dynamic in that each block (or system, or function) contributes to the strength (or development) of the others. Each system (or each building block) is mutually supporting of the others (VanSant 2005; Montgomery 2005; Bundy 2002).

This feedback loop of learning encouraging performance and performance encouraging further learning helps children to build on a skill that they already have in order to form a new skill. When this happens, children are able to form ideas about how to perform a new skill based on the foundation they have built; the foundation that was built using the sensory information received from performing a previous task. Let me give you an example of this. Children who have mastered riding a two-wheeled scooter may have an easier time learning to ride a bike. Riding a scooter takes a lot of balance and trunk stabilization to keep your body upright and midline so you don't fall over. It also requires you to use a leg to help continuously propel you. This is usually done without children ever looking at their leg to see what it is doing as they are typically looking ahead to see where they are going. This activity requires a great deal of vestibular input to maintain your balance and position in space, as well as, proprioceptive input to know what your leg is doing to help propel you, without looking it at. This vestibular and proprioceptive input received while riding the scooter has helped enhance (or build) the learning foundation through the feedback cycle that riding the scooter has given. The children can then use those skills they have developed from riding the scooter and the foundation that has been laid and apply them toward riding a bike (since riding a bike requires some of the same skills). They can form a new skill (riding a bike) using the information that they gathered, learned from, and stored in their brain while riding the scooter.

This is just one example, but it can be applied to countless other experiences. Take math, for instance. Children have to learn to count, and then recognize numbers, and then eventually learn simple addition. Once they have this foundation and information stored regarding number recognition, counting, adding, and these have become automatic skills, they can then learn subtraction. From this, they can learn more advanced math such as multiplication and division, and then eventually the big stuff like algebra and geometry! They are using their foundation to help them perform and then building their foundation bigger based on their performance and what they learn from it to help them to learn bigger and better things; it's just a big cycle!

Another example would be learning to play baseball. Children have to learn to throw and catch, then hit a stationary ball, then hit a ball in motion, etc. in order to play the game successfully. The same rules apply when learning to regulate your behaviors in a social setting. In order for children to do this, they have to learn to control their impulses, monitor their volume, hold back tears, and handle their frustrations appropriately to name a few. They also have to learn to read other's responses to their behavior through their facial expressions or reactions and adjust their behavior accordingly. This is done from the feedback received from other people's responses and then the child taking note of that, processing it, and learning from it. These skills (riding a bike, learning math, playing baseball, and learning to regulate their emotions and behaviors) are built off previous skills or experiences through the feedback loop and the foundation that was laid.

Those skills that we see at the top of the building blocks will self-organize, or come together, when children have the proper foundation. Those skills include things such as riding a bike, hitting a baseball, kicking a soccer ball, sitting still in class, focusing on work, handwriting, cutting with scissors, balancing, tolerating messy hands, controlling emotions and behaviors, etc. What is important to realize is that when there is a problem, or some dysfunction, in one of these performance areas, the first place to look is at the sensory system or the foundation of the building. The top of the building is quite dependent on the bottom of the building, and if it has not been built with a broad and firm foundation, the top of the building is at risk for toppling over.

CHAPTER 5

TURN ON THE AUTOPILOT

Studies indicate that children must develop and learn skills and habits and that child development occurs through having a big, broad base of experiences. Skills and habits are not acquired but learned.

In order for our children to develop and learn new skills, it is important to not only have a solid foundation but one that functions automatically. This will then help them to be able to focus on learning new skills rather than focusing on the basics. Athena Oden (2006) refers to this state of automatic functioning as autopilot.

> In order for our children to develop and learn new skills, it is important to not only have a solid foundation but one that FUNCTIONS AUTOMATICALLY.

What would happen if every time you drove your car you had to think about what was going on at each moment in order to keep the car running? If you had to think about the engine, transmission, carburetor, fluid levels, or the steering, accelerator, or brake systems, it would be really hard to focus on the road, let alone remember how to get to where you are trying to go. If your car is anything like mine, not only do you have to focus on where you are going but you are also trying to pop in a DVD, hand snacks to the kids, answer ten thousand questions, break up fights in the back seat, have a conversation on the cell phone, and clean up spilled milk to keep the car from stinking even worse than it already does! With all of the extraneous stuff going on in our cars while we are driving, it is a good thing that we don't have to think about the mechanics of the car; it makes driving much easier, more enjoyable, and makes getting to your destination a little safer.

While I hope that I'm not the only crazy distracted driver out there (or for safety's sake, I hope I am), I also hope you are with me in that you sometimes feel as if you are driving your car on autopilot. Sometimes I feel like I am distracted by so many other things while I am driving; yet, the next thing I know I am at my destination but don't have any idea how I got there. Does that ever happen to you?

Do you ever feel like the fact that you have driven to the same destination a million times helps you manage to get there safely without even thinking about it. It's as if the autopilot button was pressed.

Developing the sensory foundation is a lot like this. If children have to think long and hard about the basics or the mechanics, it is going to be hard for them to focus on the important stuff. Certain skills need to become automatic for children in order for them to build skills upon skills. This automatic functioning comes from thoroughly developing each of the eight senses. All of children's eight senses are interdependent on each other. If even one is not fully developed and functioning automatically, the other senses are going to suffer as well.

When skills are under children's conscious control (meaning they are still having to think about them because they are not automatic skills), they require a lot more voluntary work on their part. When skills are controlled versus being automatic, they will be performed more slowly, children will have to be more aware of what they are doing, and they will have to put more effort in to performing them. When these skills become automatic, children will perform them faster, with less conscious awareness, and with less effort.

Let's think about it for a minute. If children's vestibular and proprioceptive systems are not functioning automatically, then how are those children going to sit still in their chairs, maintain upright posture sitting in their school desk, use both hands in a coordinated way to use their scissors, or know how hard to press when writing or erasing? If the components of each of these skills are still under conscious control, they will require more effort, more awareness of what they are doing, and will be performed more slowly. This will make it hard for them to keep up with the demands placed on them in the classroom or to complete their work in a manner that is acceptable. It can also leave them flat out exhausted or ready to explode emotionally the first chance they get. If children have to put conscious thought into maintaining their equilibrium and what their body and limbs are doing, it will be very challenging to develop more complex skills. If those same children must think so hard to tune out the feel of the clothes on their body or the sound of the air conditioner kicking on or kids chattering, do you really think they are going to be able to learn to write, spell, or do math? Those things need to be automatic so that they can focus on their math or spelling. They may be able to do it, but chances are, it will be in a somewhat faulty and non-skilled manner.

I will give you an example here of something that I see a lot in the clinic that pertains to this state of autopilot. A large percentage of the children I work with have handwriting deficits. These same children more often than not also have trouble with reading and spelling. Part of the problem is that they do not have handwriting on autopilot so they have to think so hard about forming a letter that when asked to think of content to write and then spell at the same time, everything starts to crumble. Once we get the handwriting portion on autopilot so that forming their letters is done subconsciously without much thought or effort, they then have energy left to try to sound out the words and develop content for writing. Let me backup for a moment here, though. Prior to getting the skill of handwriting on autopilot, we quite frequently have to get sitting up in a chair maintaining postural control, maintaining engagement in their work, and developing motor skills to hold a pencil correctly on autopilot. You see, handwriting skills are going to be faulty every time if we don't have a foundation for the skills such as posture, focus, and pencil grip functioning automatically. Skills build off of skills and it is not until children have a good foundation and the basics functioning on autopilot that they will be able to successfully form new skills.

When we can help children gain automatic functioning of their sensory systems through the experiences we provide them, we are helping them to have the foundation off which to build new skills; therefore, we help increase their chance of success at learning new skills and building self-esteem at the same time. When the sensory system is not functioning automatically as a result of an inadequate foundation, children have to focus too much attention and put too much effort into the things that should be automatic. Consequently, children's ability to develop new and more complex skills will suffer resulting in frustration and poor self-confidence. In the same way people who are hungry have a hard time working until their hunger is satisfied, so do children whose sensory needs are not satisfied have difficulty taking on challenges that lie ahead.

CHAPTER 6

SENSORY INTEGRATION...WHAT?

The sensory foundation that we talk about is formed from our sensory experiences and the integration of the sensory stimuli we receive. As human beings, we are designed to function through the processing of the sensory input our bodies receive via its interactions with the world around us. In fact, sensory deprivation studies show that lack of sensory stimulation can actually lead to dramatic changes in the efficiency of the brain, changes that can affect memory, personality, and IQ.

Let's take a minute, then, to define sensory integration since that is what is occurring at all times as we receive information from our senses. First, let's define integration. Integration, as defined by *Merriam-Webster Dictionary*, "is the act of combining or adding parts to make a unified whole." So then **Sensory Integration** is what happens when the brain receives input from the eight senses and then uses that information efficiently and accurately to formulate a plan. It is combining, or adding, the parts (the info gathered through the senses) to make a unified whole (the whole person including emotional and behavioral regulation and motor performance). The brain must take in sensory information from the world around us, sort through and organize it, and then act on it appropriately. When this takes place as it should, it enables children to develop motor skills, regulate their emotions and behaviors, have appropriate social interactions, focus, and attend in order to learn. You can imagine, though, that with all that has to place, there is a lot of room for error.

> The BRAIN must take in sensory information from the world around us, sort through and organize it, and then act on it appropriately.

Jane Ayers, an Occupational Therapist and neuroscientist and a pioneer in the study of sensory integration, defines sensory integration as "the neurological process that organizes sensations received from one's own body and from the environment and makes it possible to use the body effectively within the environment." (Bundy, Lane, and Murray 2002). She also explained that in order to fully develop motor and cognitive skills the human brain has to internally digest and route (process) continuing feedback from all of the senses. If some of that input goes missing or is misrouted, brain circuitry becomes mixed up, and that can slow gross and fine motor maturation and delay cognitive development.

Our sensory systems are responsible for alerting our brain to potential dangers around us, as well as providing us with the opportunity to experience sensations of pleasure. Our sensory systems also allow us to realize temperature, pain, pressure, and texture and what our bodies are doing and how they are moving. Sensory integration is necessary for almost every activity that we perform because it is the combination of multiple sensory inputs that allow us to understand our surroundings. Therefore, as mentioned earlier, and we will expand upon later, motor performance (or the skills we talk about at the top of the building blocks) is greatly affected by sensory integration.

More specifically, sensory integration is the ability to take in information through our sense of movement, touch, smell, hearing, vision, and taste and then to combine that information with prior information, memories, and knowledge already stored in the brain. Combining the information that we are taking in at a given moment with the information we have gathered, stored up, learned from, and added to our foundation in the past allows us to derive meaning from the current stimuli we are experiencing. For example, we may hear a siren in the distance but can't yet see the emergency vehicle from which it is coming. Is that a police car, ambulance, or fire truck? Even though we don't see it, we recognize the sound and know we have heard it before. Oh yes, it is a fire truck. Sure enough, that fire truck soon approaches and you realize you were right. We can use our knowledge from past experiences to identify that sound despite the fact that we can't see the source. Or maybe you are reaching in your purse for a pen but are not actually looking in your purse as you feel—wallet, lipstick, Kleenex, cell phone—aha, there's the pen! You felt it because you remembered it was long and skinny, had a cap on the end, and had some textured lettering on the side. You didn't see it, but your tactile sense remembered how it felt. Your sense of touch along with your memories of how it felt helped you identify it without seeing it.

Another example of this is over a jumping over a hole in the ground. How far you jump, how much force and muscle contraction you need, how high you swing your arms to give you that extra energy you need to jump far enough, how many abdominal muscles you need to recruit for assistance, and coordinating all of this to make both feet leave the ground at the same time takes several senses all working together. Your proprioception (position), vestibular (where you are in relation to gravity), and vision senses, just to name a few, have to be working in sync to judge how far you have to jump and then make your body accommodate that. Oh wait! You had to jump almost that far another time and didn't quite make it. OK! So you need to put a little more muscle into it, swing your arms a little higher, and recruit more muscles to help you make it far enough this time.

In addition to using our foundation and prior knowledge that we have stored up to help make meaning of current stimuli, we also benefit from the fact that the information traveling to our brain is usually coming from multiple senses at one time to give us a more vivid picture of what is going on around us. For example, the use of multiple senses allows our brain to compare the information received from our auditory, visual, and vestibular system to form a complete and accurate picture of where that sound just came from in relation to where we are. *Did it come from my right or left? Is the source of the noise close to me or far away?*

The integration of our eight senses, the taking in of information, organizing it, and using it to make an appropriate response are what form our sensory foundation and, therefore, explain why opportunities to receive sensory stimuli are so important.

SECTION 2:
LET'S GET TO THE WHY

CHAPTER 7

IT'S A DIFFERENT WORLD WE LIVE IN

It is no secret that times have changed from 40, 30, 20, even 10 years ago. Things are different nowadays, and kids' behaviors are very indicative of that. Just ask any teacher trying to run and control a busy classroom. There is an increasing number of kids who can't sit still, can't focus, are impulsive, who struggle with what seems like simple activities such as going to the cafeteria, riding on the school bus, writing, or using scissors, or who just seem to stand out, but the teacher can't quite put his or her finger on the cause. Sitting in a waiting room somewhere or a restaurant and watching the number of kids playing on iphones, itouches, DS's, ipads, etc. is also indicative of changes in time.

Many of the problems or struggles our kids are dealing with can be attributed to the many changes in our society over the last 40 years. Let's face it our children have fewer opportunities to get the sensory input that they need. Without this, they will not have the broad foundation required for emotional and behavioral regulation and motor skill acquisition and mastery. Think about the days when kids left home at sunup and returned home at sundown. During that time, they were out playing. Think of all of the sensory input they received climbing trees, riding bikes, working in the fields, getting their hands dirty, etc.

> You have to LEARN To MOVE and MOVE To LEARN.

That's not how things work anymore. You have to learn to move and move to learn. Children need a tremendous number of opportunities for movement in order to learn, and this just doesn't happen these days like it used to.

Some changes, now considered technological advances, have actually had a negative effect on children's ability to build their sensory foundations. Let's take a look at some of these:

- **Survival of difficult births** – Infants now survive difficult births they may not have 40 years ago. Survival may mean a prolonged hospitalization or more time in an incubator which can decrease the amount of time they were touched, rocked, received oral input from sucking, etc., all which are vital to laying the sensory foundation. Some of the problems children face during a difficult birth (for example, a lack of oxygen to the brain) may also lead to learning or developmental delays. From my experience, I often see that twins, or an even greater number of multiples, also struggle. This could be due to premature birth, time in the NICU, or simply not having as much one-on-one time to be held, rocked, to spend on their tummies as a child who is not a multiple. Let's face it, we parents only have two arms, right?
- **The serious dangers children face** – We don't let our children just go out and run and play and ride bikes anymore. We are a lot more fearful and have to be more cautious as parents of letting our children play outside alone. I can't tell you how many times my dad has told me stories about how when he was a young boy, "I would play outside from the minute I woke up and only come home to eat dinner." I think we all agree that it seems as though we almost know too much these days and take more precautions because of this. One example of this is the fact that swings have been removed from many playgrounds for safety concerns. While that may increase safety, it decreases our children's ability to get vestibular input which is vital for laying the sensory foundation.
- **The sedentary lifestyle children experience** – Many of our children are leading a more sedentary lifestyle because they choose technology for play instead of running, jumping, climbing, and exploring their environment. Children need movement which provides all kinds of great sensory input and when they rely on TV and video games for entertainment, they are deprived of vital sensory input and their foundation suffers. Forgive me for a minute but I am going to give you the honest truth. Video games are not good for our children. In my opinion, they are the root of all evil! I cannot tell you how many children, whom I work with who, when asked what they like to do for fun, tell me "play video games." OK, so maybe they are not the root of all evil, but they do keep children from running and playing like

they should be doing and interacting with their environment in a way that will build their sensory foundation (not to mention interacting socially with their peers). Think about what children gain from watching TV. They get No interaction, No participation, No eye movement, No active concentration, and No learning how to play, create, sequence, or experiment. Sure there are programs that are educational, but they don't replace the benefits that children get from actively exploring and moving around in their environments. The fact that our children do not help with chores and heavy work around the house the way that we did as kids is another factor here. I know that in the suburb where I live a majority of families hire people to come and do their yard work or clean their houses. I know that when I was a kid those jobs belonged to my sisters and me.

- **Less tummy time as infants** – With the latest research on SIDS, our infants are sleeping on their backs and getting less time on their tummies. When infants spend time of their tummies, though, they learn so much about their world and develop equilibrium as they learn to lift their head and turn it from side to side. They learn about the weight of their limbs and gain neck and trunk strength and muscle tone. Infants have to be able to pick up their heads to actively see and learn about what is going on. Tummy time also leads to greater success with integration of their involuntary infant reflexes maturing. As I mentioned earlier, the maturation of infants' reflexes in to the voluntary movements is needed to help build their foundation. Tummy time is critical to children's development. Whether they like tummy time or not, they NEED it. Let me pause for a quick disclaimer-I **AM NOT** telling you to put your babies to sleep on their tummies. What I am saying though, is that tummy time during our infants' day is crucial to their development.

- **More time in "baby buckets"** – According to Eric Jenson, author of *Teaching with the Brain in Mind* (2005), children in 1960 spent about 200 hours in the car in their first two years of life. The average time a child spends in the car now—over 500 hours. Wow! I find that to be quite eye opening and think it says a lot. It doesn't take a rocket scientist to figure out that if our babies are spending that much time in a car, they are not getting time to lie on the floor, have tummy time, or learn to use their muscles against gravity to develop strength and muscle control. Our babies are spending so much time in "baby buckets" (and by that I mean swings, car seats, bouncy seats, etc.) and not as much time on the floor.

Think about this scenario. You need to go grocery shopping and then to the local big-box store so you can purchase diapers, formula, and other toiletries. First, you need to get dressed so you put your baby in the bouncy seat in your bedroom while you do this. Now it's time to leave, so you put your baby in the car seat and load him/her in to the car. You then pop the car seat out of the base and put it in the cart at the grocery store while you shop. After you check out at the grocery store, you pop the car seat back in to the base and drive off the local big-box store. You now pop the car seat out of the base again, place it in the stroller or the cart while you do your shopping. When you are done at that store, you pop the car seat back in to the base and head home. Oh, nice! Baby is asleep. So now you bring the car seat back into the house and let the baby take a nap in the car seat while you unload all of your groceries. Baby wakes up and needs to be fed so you take care of that then place him/her in the swing while you get dinner started.

This scenario probably spanned about 3-4 hours. That is precious time that your baby did not have any opportunities to develop any muscle strength or motor control or work on any new skills that are desperately needed to build a strong foundation for later years.

I am going to admit that this scenario is a day in the life of me with my first born. We all do what we need to do to survive. Unfortunately, this is not what is best for our children. When you were a baby, you were probably on your mom's hip a lot more during these activities. Not easy for mom, but at least it gave you the opportunity to receive sensory input because as she moved, you moved and you got to work on holding your head up against gravity and use your trunk and neck muscles to stay on her hip and not flop over. Even placing them in a sling or wrap-like carrier that is strapped to you, allows them to be upright, develop head control, and move as you move to experience vestibular input.

As I previously mentioned, the importance of tummy time for motor development, reflex maturation, and developing muscle strength and control, you can see that more time in "baby buckets" means a lot less time for development in these areas.

- **Less free play** – Let's admit it. We are all guilty of it. Every one of us parents is only trying to do what is best for our kids, but we tend to over schedule them. Having them in all kinds of managed play activities such as soccer, dance, gymnastics, etc. takes away their chance to explore and creatively manipulate their environment. I am not saying these activities are bad and there are a lot of wonderful developmental aspects to these activities. But I am saying that the majority of their playtime should be spent letting them explore and create and use their imaginations versus participating in activities where they are not given the chance to do so.

- **Technology that makes things too easy for us** – Think about the toys that you played with as a child and think about the toys your children have. While the toys our children have are fancy, light up, have all of these great sounds and buttons, many of the toys require no active participation or creativity on the children's part. The toys entertain our children rather than providing useful learning opportunities. I am going to use the example of the motorized scooter here. A large portion of the children in my neighborhood have them. I'm going to be honest, they make me cringe. While these scooters do require children to maintain their balance, they do not take much other effort on the children's behalf. These scooters are depriving children of very beneficial exercise and sensory input. Velcro shoes are another great example. Velcro shoes have made our job as parents easier but have deprived our children of learning a very valuable fine motor skill- tying shoes. To drive my point home a little more, what was your family's phone number growing up? I bet that while it could be as many as 20 plus years since you have dialed that number, you still remember it. Now, let me ask you what your parent's, friend's, or sibling's phone number is. I bet you don't know it. Speed dial and our contact lists have taken away the need for us to remember numbers. We are actually depriving our brains of a great exercise and the ability to store and recall numbers.

- **The obesity epidemic** – According to the *American Academy of Child and Adolescent Psychiatry* (2011), between 16% and 33% of children and adolescents are considered obese. The site *emedicinehealth*.com states that obesity is now one of the most widespread medical problems affecting children and adolescents in the U.S. and other developed countries and represents one of our greatest health challenges. Obesity can, of course, lead to increased health problems but also emotional and social problems. It can be a vicious cycle. Obesity, and the poor self-esteem that can come with it, can lead to depression, anxiety, and withdrawal. The emotional problems that come with obesity can then lead to further overeating, decreased activity, and increased weight gain. Overweight children will lack the energy needed to explore through active play, and therefore will feed into a more sedentary lifestyle.

John Rosemond, family psychologist, wrote in a syndicated article (1998), "Consider: In nearly every respect, what it means to be a young child has changed dramatically in the past 40 years. Alter the meaning of childhood, and you alter brain development and behavior." According to Athena Oden in *Ready Bodies, Learning Minds* (2006), we know scientifically that we learn from new experiences we have in our environment and that our brains develop from these experiences. We can gather, then, that when children (for whatever reason) have limited opportunities to experience their environment, their brain development and behavior will suffer.

Children need their days full of opportunities to move, explore with their senses, and experience their environment and for the reasons listed; many are not getting that. Children learn about their bodies through sensory feedback generated by movement. Any time we learn to do something new, any time we're confronted by a sensory stimulus that we haven't experienced before, or any time we are forced to adapt to meet the demands of the environment around us, our brain develops further.

I want to stop here, Moms, Dads, Teachers, Grandparents, etc., and say, I am not blaming or pointing fingers. Trust me, I am a mom and the last thing I want is to be made to feel as if I am doing something wrong that is causing my children to have difficulties. That is not what this book is about, so please don't take it that way. If you are reading this, then I would guarantee you are like the rest of us and just trying to do the best we know and to keep our heads above water at the same time. What I want to do is get you thinking differently. I want you to be so knowledgeable about how to provide the sensory input your children need to build their foundation that it becomes easy for you to incorporate it into their daily lives.

CHAPTER 8

THE SENSORY UMBRELLA

Through my experience, I find that by the time many parents bring their children to Occupational Therapy, they have been to just about every other specialist out there and are often just as confused as before they got started. I want to help avoid this from happening! I want you to understand that so often as parents or caregivers we exhaust ourselves worrying about every little thing our children do and exhaust ourselves trying to treat, or put a Band-Aid on, each "red flag" behavior. This does not have to be the case. Many of the problems that we see in the way our children behave or perform fall under the sensory umbrella.

When the process of taking in sensory information, organizing it, and acting on it accordingly has a kink in it, we can see a variety of problems that each need to be traced back to the sensory system. A disruption in one sensory system (i.e. the tactile, proprioceptive, or vestibular systems, etc.) is likely to affect the other sensory systems as each system is just one piece of the whole picture, and each piece is needed to make the whole picture (Remember the definition of integration adding or combining pieces to make a unified whole.). In *The Out of Sync Child* (Kranowitz 2005), Kranowitz writes, "Touch aids vision, vision aids balance, balance aids body awareness, body awareness aids movement, and movement aids learning."

An example of this is the importance of vision in maintaining balance. When I evaluate children in the clinic, I like to look at their balance and will have them stand heel to toe on a balance beam with their hands on their hips and eyes open. A majority of the time children can hold this position for an age appropriate amount of time. Next, I ask them to close their eyes. This is when the bottom drops out for many kids. They cannot keep their balance without their vision to help them. When they have to rely completely on their vestibular system in order to keep their balance, they struggle; they need their vision to help them. Each sensory system and its proper functioning is important for helping us to work like a well-oiled machine.

It is probably no surprise to you that we don't live in a perfect world, and not many of us or our children run like well-oiled machines. Most of us need a little WD-40 at times and many even need a full tune-up! When there is an immaturity or a disturbance in a sensory system, we may see many problems (that can vary greatly in severity). Below is a list of some of these problems that can fall under the sensory umbrella:

- **Attention or arousal problems** – For example, over or under arousal, difficulty focusing, or short attention span. This may also look like hypoactivity or hyperactivity.
- **Emotional or self-regulation problems** – For example, tantrums, difficulty with transitions or changes in routine, aggression toward others. You may also see low self-esteem.
- **An over or under sensitivity to sensory stimuli** – I will explain this much more in chapter 9 and then in chapter 15 as it pertains to Sensory Processing Disorder. What this means; however, is that children vary in the type and amount of sensory input they need in order for them to notice it or respond to it. They may over respond to just a little bit of stimulation or may require much more sensory input to elicit a response.
- **Difficulty discriminating sensory stimuli** – For example, discriminating between types of movement, whether or not an object is light or heavy, sharp or dull, painful or pleasurable, or discriminating between using too much or too little pressure when writing or playing with others.
- **Oculomotor/visual perceptual issues** – This includes, but is not limited to, maintaining visual focus on an object or written work, tracking a moving object with the eyes, eye fatigue, blurred vision, double vision, judging depth perception, eye-hand or eye-foot coordination, copying from the black board (or smart board), or finding a hidden object or picture amongst a group of other objects or pictures (figure-ground perception).
- **Oral issues** – For example, chewing on non-food items, being a thumb-sucker well beyond an acceptable age, gagging with textured foods, or being a picky eater.
- **Fine motor or Gross motor incoordination** – For example, difficulty using utensils or zipping zippers, fastening fasteners, tying

shoes, buttoning, catching a ball, running, skipping, jumping, etc. Motor incoordination may also make children appear clumsy.
- **Speech and language problems** – This in part goes back to the oral motor issues. For example, knowing how to move the mouth or tongue to form specific sounds (such as making the "th" sound versus the "f" sound). This also has an auditory component and affects how we process sounds around us. A large part of learning to talk is based on what we hear.
- **Weakness of the trunk or limbs/poor endurance** – Children may seem to tire easily during activities (when compared to their peers). They may have trouble holding a bat during t-ball, be unable to maneuver the monkey bars at an age when their peers can do it, slouch in their seat or always lay their heads down on their desks. They may also appear to be "double jointed" or overly flexible in their arms or legs (arms that it seems as though you could tie behind their backs).
- **Motor planning problems/difficulty in learning a new skill** – Motor planning involves creating an idea on what you want to do, formulating a plan on how to do it, and then performing the skills involved to do the task. Problems can occur in the way that children work to create the idea or in the way they execute their plan. Everything children do requires a motor plan and difficulty in this area may make it hard for them to learn a new skill and carry out motor tasks.
- **Slow processing of directions** – For example, trouble following multistep commands or instructions at all, for that matter. They may have perfect hearing but trouble processing what they hear and, therefore, difficulty following directions.
- **Difficulty at play and with forming peer relationships** – They may have trouble forming relationships with kids their age and choose to play with older or younger kids. They may tend to play by themselves and rarely interact with other children during play dates, at the park, in the classroom, etc.
- **Learning challenges** – These problems listed above can spill over into the classroom as children may have trouble learning math, reading, writing, etc. When children have to work so hard in these other areas, it makes it very difficult to focus their attention on the actual learning side of school.

CHAPTER 9

THE SENSORY CUPS

I mentioned in the previous chapter that one of the problems we may see in our children that fall under the sensory umbrella is an over and undersensitivity to sensory input. I want to spend a little more time explaining that because every one of us has over and undersensitivity when it comes to various sensory stimuli. Somebody would have a hard time convincing me that they didn't. However, the degree to which our sensitivities affect us vary.

As I talk about sensory cups please keep in mind that I am simplifying this to help give you a basic understanding, and the example of cups I am using is certainly not scientific in nature.

We all require a certain amount of water to keep us hydrated and keep our bodies running properly. We also have different preferences for what we choose to drink to keep us hydrated. Some of us simply choose water while others may prefer a sports drink and others choose some of these fancy flavored waters enhanced with all kinds of different vitamins and minerals. Some of us will chug the whole thing quickly and others prefer to sip on their drink for hours. Some of us put a few ounces in our cup knowing this will fill us up and others pour the whole 16 ounces in their cup knowing they can drink this much in one big gulp without filling up.

In the same way that our bodies need hydration, our brains need sensory input to maintain proper function. We differ; however, in how much we can fill our cup and tolerate before we are full. The amount of fluid needed in our cup to satisfy our thirst and fill us up can be compared to how much sensory input is needed to help us reach and maintain our optimum level of arousal. I will explain in much greater detail the optimum level of arousal in chapter 10, but for now it is important to understand that this is the level at which children will be best able to focus, attend, interact with peers, learn, etc.

Some children have a very small cup and cannot tolerate much fluid in theirs before it overflows. This is similar to children with sensory oversensitivity. Children who have small cups can become overloaded from sensory input quite easily; it doesn't take much. If these children's cups are filled too full, they will become over reactive to sensory stimulation and you may see troubling behaviors because of it. When this happens they may seem anxious, fearful, or uncomfortable from sensory stimuli that other children seem to tolerate without any trouble. They may exhibit a "fight, flight, or fright" response, meaning that they will shut down to avoid the situation, try to escape the situation, or become aggressive in response to being in a state of sensory overload. Things such as getting their hands dirty, trying a new food, being in a loud movie theater, or going to a birthday party at the pizza place with singing and dancing animals on stage are just a few examples of situations that may cause their cup to overflow.

The opposite also exists. There are children who seem to have a two liter bottle from which to drink, and it takes a lot of fluid to fill them up. These children are under-sensitive to sensory input; consequently, it takes a lot more of that input for them to perceive it and respond to it. It takes a lot of fluid to quench their thirst and get them to their optimum level of arousal. When their cups (or two liters) are not filled up, they are left "thirsty" and will act accordingly. In my experience, I have seen a variety of behaviors associated with this. I have seen children who seem withdrawn, tuned out, or oblivious because they have not received enough "fluid" in their cup for them to seem aware or respond to the sensory stimulation. I have also seen children who will work to get more sensory input in an attempt to fill their cup and reach their optimum level of arousal; these children, for example, may constantly be on-the-go and can't seem to be still.

There can be thousands of combinations of over and undersensitivities of the eight senses. For example, a combination of oversensitivity with some of the eight senses and undersensitivity with other senses may look something like this: Imagine, for example, a young boy, let's call him Sam, who reacts negatively to touch, does not like to get his hands dirty, and is a picky eater. Sam may also have a hard time sitting still and focusing in the classroom, and at home he is always on the go and never seems to sit down. Sam may have a dislike of crowds and may tend to avoid situations where he will have to be in one. In fact, the last time he left a loud birthday party, he came home and had a complete meltdown.

Sam is demonstrating a tactile oversensitivity, meaning that his tactile cup reaches its brim very easily, therefore, causing him to avoid situations involving touch and textures. Sam is also demonstrating a vestibular undersensitivity in that he needs movement to focus. His vestibular cup does not get filled to the point where an optimum level of arousal will be reached by simply sitting still in his desk. He needs movement (and lots of it) to fill his sensory cup to the level where he will feel ready to focus. Sam's dislike and avoidance of crowds also shows us that he may have an auditory oversensitivity, and the noise from crowds may cause his cup to overflow. The fact that loud (and typically very overstimulating) birthday parties cause him to have a meltdown drives home the fact that his sensory cup overflowed and now we see the emotional and behavioral breakdown because of it.

You may be wondering why your children (or even you) have cups that overflow quickly or two liters that can't get filled up. The first thing to know is that it is neurological in nature. It is because the brain is not filtering the amount and intensity of sensory information that it is processing. What happens then is our children have a hard time modulating (adapting to a certain proportion or regulating) that sensory information. When children have a hard time adapting to or regulating the sensory information that they receive, it will manifest itself as oversensitivites and undersensitivities.

Again, we all have a cup or two that needs more to fill it or that overflows fairly easily whether we realize it or not. This is OK. Once you understand this, it may help you understand your children's behavior a little more and then help you know how to respond appropriately. The key is to learn to read what your children are trying to tell you through their actions, responses, behaviors, etc. and realize what it is that they need more or less of. Once you realize this, you will be better equipped to help them. It is when it starts to cause problems in children's daily function that we start to worry a little and need to speak to their physician and seek out Occupational Therapy.

> The kEY is to learn to read what your children are trying to tell you through their actions, responses, behaviors, etc. and realize what it is that they need more or less of.

CHAPTER 10

OPTIMUM LEVEL OF AROUSAL AND SELF-REGULATION

I want to take this time to define this term optimum level of arousal that I keep mentioning. Children's optimum level of arousal is closely linked to their sensory system and is a key factor in self-regulation (or their ability to regulate their emotional and behavioral responses to sensory stimulation). Arousal is the state of being alert, awake, attentive and reactive to sensory stimulation. Arousal can refer to how much capacity you have available to work with. Arousal is important in regulating consciousness, attention, memory, processing information, and is crucial for regulating certain behaviors. The optimum level of arousal then, is a state of being at that "just right" level of alertness in order for children to perform at their best. The "just right" amount can motivate children, but too much or too little arousal will hamper their performance. Certain tasks can require certain arousal levels as well. Being overly aroused may be good on the ball field but not in algebra class and vice versa.

> The optimum level of arousal then, is a state of being at that "JUST RIGHT" level of alertness in order for children to perform at their best.

Arousal level and responsiveness to sensory information (by that I mean the over or undersensitivity that I talked about in the chapter 9) are physiologically different but can often go hand in hand. When children are overly sensitive to the sensory input they are receiving, you will often find them to be overly aroused (or overly reactive to sensory stimulation). When they are under-sensitive to sensory input, they will often appear to be under aroused (or under reactive to sensory stimulation). How children choose to deal with their arousal level is what can sometimes throw up some red flags to us as caregivers. As I have mentioned, over or under arousal will have a negative impact on their ability to attend, their ability to process the information they are receiving, and their performance and can then impair their ability to function successfully in their daily activities.

Optimum level of arousal refers to our ability to maintain an optimal level of performance and an optimum level of alertness that will allow us to focus, attend, and complete the tasks being required of us. Self-regulation is the ability to change our arousal level or maintain the arousal level that is necessary to meet the demands of the task or situation. Self-regulation, then, is our ability to achieve and sustain an optimum arousal level - aroused enough to function but not too aroused to focus or to control our behaviors and emotions. As adults we may tap our foot, drink cold water or hot coffee, chew gum, bite our nails, pace, etc. to self-regulate or get our arousal level where it needs to be to focus on an instructor, sit through a long meeting, or keep us awake when driving.

> SELF-REGULATION is the ability to change our arousal level or maintain the arousal level that is necessary to meet the demands of the task or situation.

Regulating the arousal level begins at birth and is critical in order for children to adapt to a constantly changing environment. Have you ever heard of babies who were extremely fussy or colicky, picky with foods or the manner in which they were fed, hated to be on their tummies, cried all the time, and were very particular about things such as their car seat or swing, or how they were held? If so, then you have heard of (or perhaps had one of your own) someone who had trouble self-regulating even as an infant. At the advice of my son's pediatrician when he was an infant, we did not try to discourage him from sucking his thumb or pacifier. What he was actually doing when he sucked his thumb or his pacifier was self-regulating. When babies suck their thumbs or a pacifier or have a favorite "lovey" or "blankie," that is not always bad. They are soothing themselves or self-regulating.

Our children need to learn how to use these techniques for themselves and some children need more help with this than others. Children will often choose what we find to be inappropriate ways to self-regulate. Under aroused children may seek out input by biting their shirt, chewing their fingernails, fidgeting, squirming in their seat, etc. in an attempt to self-regulate. Overly aroused children may throw tantrums or have a meltdown in their own attempt to self-regulate. Children struggling with their sensory system and their sensory foundation may require extra help to reach an optimum arousal level and find appropriate ways in which to do so. These children require a lot of instruction and cueing as to how they can begin to do this for themselves.

Arousal, then, is not only important in regulating our attention and the ability to process information, but is also very closely tied with self-regulation and emotional and behavioral control. Let's think about the emotions or behaviors we may exhibit when we are not at our optimum level of arousal. How do you respond when you are overly aroused? How do you feel mentally when your co-workers are pulling you in different directions, when you hear "Mom, Mom, Mom, Mom, Mom" over and over, after an afternoon with the kids at that pizza place with lots of video games and singing robotic animals on stage, or when you simply just have a lot on your mind? You may get real fidgety, have a hard time sitting still and focusing on the task in front of you, be quick to anger or to lose your patience, be really excitable, or feel like you need to shut down or jump out of your skin.

Now think about when you are under aroused. I would venture to say most of our arousal levels differ greatly from a Monday morning to a Friday afternoon. Talk to me pre-coffee on a Monday morning and it will not seem as though I am conscious or ready to process anything; I am under aroused (or under reactive to stimuli). After some coffee, bring it on! When we are feeling really tired or lazy (think of a rainy Sunday afternoon), it may be hard to focus, concentrate, listen and comprehend, or make sense of what is going on. It may be difficult to make any big decisions or have the motivation to get up and take on a challenging task. If you are someone who likes to exercise in the morning, think about why and how it makes you feel afterwards. Exercising gets you going. It gets your engine running, your mind focused, and gives you energy to conquer your day. It helps you get to your optimum level of arousal.

Our kids experience these same problems just in different ways. It is important to be able to read their arousal level and make the appropriate accommodations. If children are in a state of under or overarousal, chances are sitting to focus on a math test or spelling words is going to be very challenging. When we can determine their arousal level, we can choose activities to help bring that level up or down (whichever is needed) to achieve an optimum level of arousal. Perhaps they need to stand up and do some jumping jacks, toe touches, spin in circles, or listen to music to increase their level of arousal, or maybe they need some calming strategies to be put in place to decrease their level of arousal.

Difficulty with self-regulation can also make it difficult for children to "shift-gears", making transitions quite difficult. Transitioning to an awake state after sleeping or transitioning to bedtime after a full day, transitioning home after school or to school from the school bus, and transitioning from one activity to another can be challenging. When we understand our children's sensory cups and how they relate to their arousal level, we can help them develop strategies to get through these situations. These strategies include sensory activities to calm over-responsive children who have reached a state of overarousal. In addition, we may have to use strategies to bring alertness to under-responsive children who appear to be under aroused or help them to fill their cups in an appropriate way. As you continue to read you will gain an understanding of what strategies you can use with your children.

CHAPTER 11

THE IMMATURE SENSORY SYSTEM

Let's face it. Most of our children struggle to some degree in one way or another. Growing and developing is not for the faint of heart. Some struggle with their ability to self-regulate. Some struggle to focus on their school work. Others have "quirky" behaviors that we just don't understand. And some appear clumsy or seem to be lagging behind their peers when it comes to their motor skills. Hopefully, you are starting to realize that many of their struggles go back to their foundation and their sensory system.

You may be like so many of the parents with whom I speak with who are worried there is a "problem", or who are looking for a "diagnosis" to help explain their worrisome behaviors. I feel that sometimes when there is a label or diagnosis it helps us to feel like we can find a recipe to fix the problem. Often children get diagnosed with a developmental delay (such as a speech, fine motor, or gross motor delay) which can be rooted in the sensory system. There are also several diagnoses available that involve problems with sensory integration and sensory processing including Sensory Processing Disorder, ADD/ADHD, and autism spectrum disorder. What I want to introduce you to is the concept of the immature sensory system because I feel this is getting to be a bigger and bigger problem in our society. Our children may not always require a medical diagnosis; what our children are really showing are signs of an immature sensory system.

Let me start by explaining an **immature sensory system**. The definition of immature is something that is not fully developed. Therefore, an immature sensory system is a sensory system that is not fully developed. That doesn't mean there is a "problem" per se, or that the child needs a label. What it does mean is that the sensory system needs help to mature (or fully develop). When children's

> When children's sensory systems are NOT MATURE, chances are you will see problems in areas of performance and emotional/behavioral regulation.

sensory systems are not mature, chances are you will see problems in areas of performance and emotional/behavioral regulation.

This may show up as learning difficulties, poor attention span, poor impulse control, emotional immaturity, difficulty with motor skills and coordination, eating and speech problems, and hyperactivity.

A study done by the Sensory Processing Disorder Scientific Work Group (Ben-Sasson, Carter, Briggs-Gowen 2009) suggests that one in every six children experience sensory symptoms that are significant enough to affect their everyday life. I believe the number is even higher; however, when you take into account the number of children who struggle with an immature sensory system. They may not experience sensory symptoms great enough to have a huge impact on their day-to-day function, but there's enough going on to know there's something that seems a little off. I believe that many children these days do not have the sensory foundation needed to fully evolve their sensory processing system. Not having a good sensory foundation and problems with processing sensory information can then lead to problems either in the way the brain receives information, the way it organizes it, the way children formulate a motor plan to carry out a certain task, or the way children respond emotionally or behaviorally.

Formulated from my years of experience as an Occupational Therapist combined with current research, I do not feel all children need or warrant a diagnosis. Now let me stop and emphasize how important it is to consult the children's doctor and an Occupational Therapist when you see them struggling at the top of the building blocks (motor skills/performance and emotional and behavioral regulation) when it is interfering with their daily life, but I want to urge you to start by looking at the sensory system. What I find so often is that many of the problems children are having that have led their parents in all sorts of different directions to get help, fall under one umbrella of a problem; a problem with their sensory foundation. As stated by Athena Oden in *Ready Bodies, Learning Minds* (2006), attention to immature development can be a first step in early prevention of school failure.

We all have our sensory quirks or things to which we are overly-sensitive or under-sensitive. Many of us have a hard time sitting still and feel the need to fidget, tap our pencil, chew our pen cap or our nails when stressed or trying to concentrate. Many of us are sensitive to loud noises or are picky eaters. We get by though. We have learned that there are things we can do to compensate when we are under stimulated (for example, drink caffeine, exercise, or get up and move around) or find ways to avoid the things that we know will get us overstimulated (for example, limit our outings to the pizza place with the dancing mouse and bears). Many of our children have the same sensory quirks; they just haven't figured out how to cope with them yet. What I want to help you do is identify the behaviors that you see in your children, determine which one of the senses they fall under, and give you ideas on ways to give your children the boost they need to that sensory system.

So, "Why do children have immature sensory systems?" you may ask. A lot of it has to do with the changes in our society over the last 40 years—kids not playing outside as much, time on screens, and the demands of our society that keep us and our families overscheduled—play a big role in the underdeveloped sensory system.

It is my opinion that the immature sensory system is exacerbated by the demands that are placed on our children these days. I am going to ask for forgiveness in advance, but I am about to get on my soap box for a moment. I believe that with the increased demands on our kids in school, with all of the extracurricular activities they are involved in, the changes in our society over the last 40 years, and the fact that we are asking them to not only perform, but succeed at things at a much younger age than we were asked, we are putting our kids at risk. We are putting them at risk of not being able to keep up with the demands placed on them academically, at home, and in extracurricular activities. We are putting them at risk of failure in school, on the ball field, and in forming meaningful relationships with their peers. We are putting them at risk of developing a poor self-esteem, shutting down or acting up, and having a label placed on them as a result. While a diagnosis is warranted for some children and proper diagnosis is vital for treatment, let's start by looking at the sensory system.

When I was in kindergarten, we still had nap time, we had three recesses, and we were learning our ABC's. I don't think we started in organized sports until we were at least eight years old. Now in kindergarten, children are expected to sit and attend for up to an eight-hour-day without much time for recess and running around (the things that help neurologically organize children the most for learning), write full sentences, complete homework after a long day of school, and then participate in extracurricular activities after school and on the weekends. Wow! That is a lot of pressure on five-or-six-year-olds. As a clinician, I work with a lot of kindergarteners who are struggling to keep up with demands placed on them. Their teachers often realize these children stand out amongst their peers because of their behaviors or because of what they can't do and have recommended some outside help. What I find is that often these children have immature sensory systems and that their sensory foundations aren't big enough and now the stress of kindergarten and the demands placed on them really start to become apparent.

I remember when my son started kindergarten. My husband and I decided to give him an extra year because he has a summer birthday, so he started at the age of six years and two months. I have already mentioned to you that he is a "typically" developing child but definitely has his share of sensory quirks. I observed firsthand the stress that kindergarten can place on a child. In the first month of school, he learned so much academically that it blew my mind (and kind of brings tears to my eyes as a proud mom when I think about it). He was learning "sight words," learning addition and subtraction, learning to sound words out, read, and to write stories. He also had to learn how to sit in an extremely loud cafeteria with a few hundred kids and eat his lunch without anyone to remind him to eat his fruit first. He had to learn to pack and unpack his book bag all by himself. He had to learn to be responsible for his things, to keep his chair pushed in, raise his hand when he wanted to talk instead of blurting something out, and how to make friends with a whole new group of kids. He also had to build up his endurance to tolerate a seven-hour-day, five days a week. Oh my goodness! We probably should have held him back another year and waited until he was seven. That is a lot! No wonder it makes me tear up!

Now, while my son was doing well in school, I saw what this was doing to his foundation. When he got off of the school bus in the afternoon, I could tell right away by looking at him how the rest of our evening was going to go. After holding it together all day at school, as soon as he saw the face of someone who would unconditionally love him, he broke down as he was finally able to let it all go after holding it together all day long. He was also doing things that showed me that his sensory foundation was struggling and needed another boost. He was putting things in his mouth a lot (which he had never done before), he tugged on his shirt constantly as if to readjust it on his body, had more meltdowns (over practically nothing), he was harder to rationalize with and became much more stubborn, he fidgeted constantly and couldn't sit still (even to watch his favorite TV show). He was seeking out rougher play at home by jumping on furniture, pushing heavy things around, and wrestling (quite roughly) with my husband.

The point I am trying to make here is that even my "typically" developing son, was obviously feeling the stress of the demands of kindergarten and was acting in ways I had never seen him act before. Was I worried about him? No. What I did was read from what his actions were telling me he needed and helped to strengthen his sensory foundation. What had happened was that his nice little building blocks of learning with a good broad foundation had taken a hit. That foundation needed some re-edifying because this storm called kindergarten had chipped away at it. I made sure he had plenty of free time after school to ride his bike, swing, run around with the neighbor kids, jump, climb, etc. If it was a rainy day, I made sure we did a lot of activities inside that would give him vestibular and proprioceptive input. I made sure his structured activities were at a minimum (one extracurricular activity and that is it). I gave him a great deal of opportunities for heavy work since he is showing me by jumping, wrestling, and playing rough that he needed that. I gave him deep pressure input by rolling a ball down his back frequently. I made sure he used his punching bag as much as possible. I made sure his meals consisted of chewy and crunchy foods. By doing this and rebuilding his building blocks before too much damage was done, I was able to help him have more confidence that he could face the demands placed on him. (Don't worry; I will talk a lot more about these activities in the chapters to come.)

Often, we realize our children may have some minor struggles or sensory quirks (For example, they can't hold their pencil right, can't seem to get the hang of dressing themselves, have difficulty learning to throw and catch, seem emotionally immature, or seem a bit clumsy.) Well. OK. Hopefully they will outgrow it. Right? Hopefully they will, but put those children in kindergarten (or any other stressful situation) with lots of demands on their sensory system and you will likely find that what you thought they would outgrow is now getting even worse. This happens at every grade level—not just in kindergarten. When children's sensory foundations are not firm enough, we tend to see problems get bigger and bigger as they get older and the stressors placed on them increase (instead of outgrowing them as we had hoped).

What I am trying to convey here, and I will get off my soap box soon, is that our kids need help to outgrow their struggles or quirks, and they need help to learn to compensate for them. Just because children are struggling handling the demands placed on them doesn't necessarily mean they have a "problem" or need to be medicated. These children need to build their sensory foundation. The great news is that it is never too late to start, and, like most things, the sooner the better. If these children are exposed to all kinds of great sensory stimulation to enhance their sensory processing abilities, it will help with motor planning and execution abilities. They will have a better understanding, through these experiences, of how to integrate all of the senses they are utilizing at any given moment and understand how to act on them and use their bodies appropriately. ALL children can benefit from activities to enhance and mature their sensory foundation, whether they seem to be struggling in a few areas with a few sensory quirks or developing right on track.

CHAPTER 12

THE PROPRIOCEPTIVE (PRO-PRI-O-CEP-TIVE) SYSTEM

I feel I need to pause briefly here and refer you to chapter 20 if you are feeling the slightest bit stressed, overwhelmed, or wondering if there is any hope. In that chapter I share with you that our brains have what is called neuroplasticity. This amazing feature allows our brains to change, develop, learn, and mature. So stick with me because you are going to become an expert at performing plastic surgery on your child's brain.

Now let me get back to where I was. To ensure that you have a good understanding of the proprioceptive system, refer back briefly to chapter 2 where I described the proprioceptive system in more detail. I mentioned in that chapter that the proprioceptive system gives us our sense of position. It helps us to understand our movements with the proprioceptive receptors being in our joints and ligaments. Proprioceptive information is gathered when we stretch or contract our muscles or bend, straighten, pull, or compress our joints. This system plays a large role in our body awareness, motor control, motor planning, and posture. This system tells our brain where our bodies are in relation to our surroundings and other objects and then tells our bodies how to move efficiently. The proprioceptive system helps us with things such as knowing if our elbow is bent or straight (without having to look at it), knowing if we are squeezing something hard or gently, being able to run quickly and walk smoothly, and allows us to keep our eyes on the road while riding our bikes or driving instead of watching what our arms, hands, and feet are doing.

Before I talk about what it may look like when children do not have the proprioceptive foundation that they need, I want to mention briefly one reason *why* we may be seeing an increase in the number of children who have an immature proprioceptive system. Our society does not lend itself, these days, to providing children with opportunities for heavy work (or proprioceptive input). Think about

THE PROPRIOCEPTIVE (PRO-PRI-O-CEP-TIVE) SYSTEM

the generations before ours. I think about my parents who were born in the late 40's early 50's and the generations before them. They played outside all day, worked on the farm, played pick-up basketball or kickball in the street or local playground, rode bikes everywhere they went, and walked to school with heavy backpacks. Apparently, both of my parents had to walk uphill both ways to school in snow up to their eyeballs. Furthermore, they had summer jobs involving manual labor, had a large responsibility completing household chores, and so on.

REMEMBER: You have to LEARN To MOVE and MOVE To LEARN!

Our kids don't do those things. Therefore, they do not get the opportunities for their bodies to benefit from proprioceptive input. Playing video games, sitting at the computer, and watching TV do not lend themselves to opportunities for proprioceptive input or heavy work. Because of these factors, our kids are missing out on opportunities to build their strength, postural stability, and sensory foundation. As a result, you may see children seeking out proprioceptive input in ways that seem confusing or alarming to you. Once again, the key is to realize *why* they are doing what they are doing.

Some children may struggle with the information that they receive from their proprioceptive receptors. When this happens, some children will seek out more intense forms of proprioceptive input. They need more of it to achieve their optimum level of arousal. The reason is that our bodies should receive enough proprioceptive input at rest to let our brain feel secure about what our bodies are doing so we can take our minds off of our body and focus it elsewhere. When children are inefficiently integrating the sensations that they get from their muscles and joints, they do not register enough input just through maintaining their posture or upright position against gravity; therefore, they require more input to do so.

What does this look like? Children with this characteristic will need to increase the amount or intensity of input their proprioceptive system is getting in order to give their brain the information it needs so they can feel secure about what their body is doing in space. They will find ways to load their proprioceptive receptors through heavy work, chewing on things, playing too rough, squeezing too hard, moving, jumping, fidgeting, etc. They need movement, resistance, pressure, and lots more of it to get their brains to an optimal level of

> The proprioceptive system gives us our SENSE OF POSITION.

arousal and to feel secure enough about what their bodies are doing to be able to turn their focus elsewhere (for instance to focus on their schoolwork).

An immature or dysfunctional proprioceptive system may also cause children to have trouble with planning their movements, controlling their movements, and with body awareness (or understanding what their bodies are doing). This, again, goes back to the fact that they are not receiving correct information from their proprioceptive receptors about what their bodies are doing. Without the correct information and not knowing how much stretch, pull, contraction, bend, etc. they are getting to the muscles, joints, and ligaments, they may seem clumsy, have difficulty with fine motor and gross motor skills, have difficulty sitting upright in their desk without slouching, or have difficulty "grading" their movements (knowing how much force or speed to use and whether to use big or small movements).

When the proprioceptive system is not running smoothly, children will have difficulty modulating the proprioceptive information that they receive or struggle because they are not correctly processing the information that they receive from their muscles, joints, and ligaments. It can manifest itself in a variety of ways:

Seeking out proprioceptive input

- **Large and fast movements** – These children will often use big movements for most activities. It takes big movements for them to register that they are moving. In addition to this, big movements require less motor control. An example of this would be children who use their whole body to throw a ball or, when hopping on one leg, have to hold their opposite leg way up in the air as if they are bracing themselves.
- **Seek out heavy work** – They may love to carry, push, or pull heavy items. The more resistance and the heavier, the better. Some examples of this that I have seen in the clinic are a four-year-old boy who loved to vacuum (Think about how heavy of work that is for a four-year-old.) and would come to see me with a backpack filled with about ten-pounds worth of canned goods. I saw another kid who loved heavy work so he would move furniture around the house and insisted on physically pushing his parents out of the door when they were leaving him (in a loving way, though). My own daughter loves to hang on her elbows from the kitchen table when eating vs. sitting in a chair. She needs to use big muscles in order to focus on eating. Just sitting on a chair at the table won't do it.

THE PROPRIOCEPTIVE (PRO-PRI-O-CEP-TIVE) SYSTEM

- **Seek out jumping activities** – Often these kids could jump on a trampoline for days if no one stopped them. They will often find any way to work jumping in to their day whether it be jumping on furniture or beds, jumping down from high places, or just jumping while standing in line. A great example of this is a young boy who loved jumping so much that he would jump on his mini indoor trampoline while playing video games or would simply jump up and down on the ground while standing in line with his mom at the store.
- **Chew on non-food items or grind their teeth** – When we chew, we get heavy work to our oral musculature. Often kids will chew on their shirts, pens, fingers, bubble gum, etc. to use those heavy muscles. I have seen children bite others to receive this same proprioceptive input (which is obviously a troublesome situation, but once we figure out *why* they are doing this we can channel this need appropriately). These children will often have wet shirt collars. I have been in preschools where kids are trying so hard to stay in the line and walk quietly to the classroom and all you hear from the teachers is "Get your shirts out of your mouths." Chances are the children are trying so hard to control themselves and follow the rules of being quiet and walking slowly that they need to chew their shirts to help them stay on task and stay focused on following the rules.
- **Love roughhousing or "squishing" activities** – These children will love to tackle and be tackled, or to squeeze or be squeezed. The rougher the play the better because it will give them deep pressure or more intense proprioceptive input. The same little boy who loved to vacuum and carried a ten-pound backpack wanted his mom to wrestle with him constantly. He would come straight in to the clinic and head for the weighted balls or a ball pump that he would want to pump our whole session (Think of how much muscle it takes to pump a ball or pump.). Other kids love it when I put a bean bag chair on top of them and then (gently) lie on top of it. They will request this activity because of the input the "squishing" gives them.
- **Seem to enjoy falling and do it for no reason** – When we fall on the ground, we receive lots of proprioceptive input from the impact of our bodies hitting the ground. I have worked with kids who, after every movement they performed, would fall to the ground.

- **Fidgeter** – Are your children constantly moving their leg up and down, tapping their pencil on their desk, twirling their hair with their fingers, or fidgeting with something in their hand? These activities are often done subconsciously by children in an effort to increase their ability to focus. By fidgeting they get increased proprioceptive input and awareness of what their bodies are doing. Without that input or awareness, they feel insecure about their bodies and have to focus so much energy on figuring out what their bodies are doing that they don't have enough energy left to focus on the task at hand.
- **Tiptoe walking** – Walking on tippy-toes can be seen as proprioceptive or tactile dysfunction (You will see this again in the tactile chapter.). One explanation for tiptoe walking is that children receive more proprioceptive input by walking on their tiptoes than on the balls of their feet. A woman who has high-functioning autism and who created the website "Autism and Its World" describes tiptoe walking this way: "When autistic people walk on their toes, it is because it provides a greater sense of 'feeling your body and knowing where it is in space' and helps balance and feeling like you're not going to tip over."

Signs of poor body awareness and motor control
- **Use too much or too little force or pressure** – These kids will have difficulty grading their movements and will stomp their feet, slam doors, squeeze and break Styrofoam cups or toys, etc. all because they can't judge how much pressure or force to use, therefore they use too much. To them they are putting their books down on their desk slowly and gently, when in reality, they just slammed them down on their desk. We often see this in writing when kids who use too much pressure writing or erasing.
- **Weak muscles** – These kids are not registering proprioceptive input appropriately in a way that will "wake-up" their muscles. They will seem to be weak especially when compared to their peers. This is often noticed during athletics or playground activities such as climbing or trying to make it across the monkey bars.
- **Slump, lean, or prop themselves** – In order to feel stable, these kids will prop themselves by leaning on walls or furniture, lay their heads on their desks, or slump in their seats. These actions actually take proprioception (or having to know what their bodies are doing) out of

THE PROPRIOCEPTIVE (PRO-PRI-O-CEP-TIVE) SYSTEM

the equation so they can focus on their schoolwork or the task at hand vs. having to spend the energy trying to figure out what their bodies are doing.

- **Poor body awareness** – These kids will have difficulty understanding what their bodies are doing or what space they occupy compared to the world around them.
- **Appear clumsy** – Without proper feedback about your body and its movements, coordinated movements will be difficult. When children have trouble grading their movements they may misjudge how much force or speed to use often knocking things over making them appear clumsy.

This list is not all-inclusive, but I wanted to give you an idea of what our proprioceptive system does and what it may look like when this system is not functioning properly. If you realize that your children may be struggling with an immature proprioceptive system or have proprioceptive dysfunction, you can then figure out what to do for them and know how to fill their days with opportunities to help mature their sensory system.

When children have a proprioceptive dysfunction, it can make life very challenging. Just trying to accomplish what may seem like a normal everyday activity can be hard. Because of this, they may suffer emotionally and lack self-confidence and avoid trying new things or playing like typical kids play. Make sure you seek out the advice and guidance of an Occupational Therapist if you feel your children are struggling in this way.

I mentioned in chapter 2 that proprioceptive input can be both calming and neurologically organizing. What this means is that it can help children organize all of the other sensory information they are receiving from the world around them. It can increase their alertness, decrease their anxiety, can counter sensory over sensitivities, and help children get their brains prepped and ready to go (in other words, help them focus). This is very important to remember as you will want to make sure you have a big bag of proprioceptive tricks readily available to you to help your children when you see they need it. When in doubt, give your child proprioceptive input!

> When in doubt, give your child PROPRIOCEPTIVE INPUT!

Refer to chapter 23 for a list of activities that you can do with your child to build their proprioceptive system.

CHAPTER 13

THE VESTIBULAR (VES-TIB-U-LAR) SYSTEM

The next sensory system that we want to look at more in depth is the vestibular system. To ensure that what I am about to say will make sense, please briefly refer back to chapter 2 where I described the vestibular system in more detail.

Just to recap; however, the vestibular system is important for the development of balance, postural control, muscle tone, coordination, eye control, focusing and maintaining attention, and feeling secure about and tolerating movement.

The vestibular system is located in the inner ear and, through the position and movement of our heads, tells our brains where our bodies are in relationship to the rest of the world. Vestibular information helps us to determine the direction and speed of movement and gives us an understanding of up and down, fast and slow, right and left, etc.

It is because of its location in the inner ear that the vestibular system is involved in some aspects of auditory processing and language development. This system's nerves actually run in close connection to the nerves that are dedicated to hearing (the cochlear nerves). I point this out as a side note because the implications, then, are that when working with children with speech deficits, we can boost their ability to improve in this area by also boosting their vestibular system.

> The VESTIBULAR SYSTEM is located in the inner ear and, through the position and movement of our heads, tells our brains where our bodies are in relationship to the rest of the world.

There is something else we should think of as a result of the vestibular system's close connection with the cochlear (hearing) system. Because of this system's location, it is speculated that children with a history of chronic ear infections may also exhibit signs of vestibular dysfunction. The reason for this is that when children have an ear infection, the brain is getting inconsistent and possibly incorrect messages. This can cause the brain to raise its threshold for vestibular input; therefore, requiring more than the normal amount of input to be needed for the vestibular system to respond. I mention this because the children with whom I work who exhibit an immature vestibular system or vestibular dysfunction quite commonly have had a history of ear infections as an infant and required PE tubes to be placed (not to say that the two always go hand in hand, however).

When the vestibular system is not functioning smoothly, it can become difficult for children to modulate vestibular input and to get their sensory cup filled to that "just right" level. Children who are under-sensitive to vestibular input just can't seem to get their sensory cup filled up to the point where they will be at the optimum level of arousal. Just like with the proprioceptive system, children who are under-sensitive to vestibular input can respond in different ways. They may seem as if they do not get pleasure from movement, therefore, preferring sedentary activities and lacking participation in physical activities (such as sports, gym, and activities that involve running, jumping, swinging, or climbing). Under-sensitive children may also appear to seek out vestibular input in an attempt to fill their cup. They do not register enough input by just sitting still and holding themselves up against gravity so they work to increase the amount that they get. These children will move constantly to get more vestibular information in order to fill their cup, and they may seek out intense forms of movement.

Children who are over-sensitive to vestibular input tend to have their sensory cup filled up quickly requiring only a minimal amount of input to do so. They tend to reach a state of over-stimulation (or overarousal) very quickly; it doesn't take much. Because of this they may be fearful of and avoid activities that require their feet to leave the ground (for example, climbing, swinging, or riding a bike). These children will often have poor balance (especially with their eyes closed), have difficulty standing on one foot, and may appear clumsy.

The vestibular system helps to maintain our arousal through its connection to the Reticular Activating System (RAS). The RAS is the alerting system of the brain and helps keep us responsive to sensory stimuli. The RAS also acts as a screening device to help us determine what incoming sensory information is important and what is not. This system helps to wake us up and increases our excitability and responsiveness to stimulation through activating the "fight, flight, or fright" system. When children have an imbalance in their RAS and their vestibular system, it can cause them to be "on edge" and overreact to stimuli. This may then cause children to overreact to vestibular input creating a situation where more vestibular input will cause them to become more hyperactive and disorganized. This is important to know because some children (even those who appear to seek out vestibular input) can become increasingly hyper with vestibular input. When you see this occur, you have to realize that you need to reduce the intensity, frequency, duration, etc. of the vestibular input and be sure to follow any vestibular input with proprioceptive input which is calming and organizing input.

When things are not running smoothly with the vestibular system, like the other systems, children will have a hard time reaching and maintaining an optimum level of arousal and modulating the sensory input that they receive. Characteristics of an immature vestibular system or vestibular dysfunction can manifest itself along a wide spectrum. Below is a list of behaviors or problems you may see with an immature vestibular system or vestibular dysfunction:

Under-sensitive to vestibular input

- **In constant motion** – Does it seem like your children can't sit still? Some children need more motion to activate their vestibular system and until they do so, they do not feel secure and will struggle to focus and attend. The information gathered through simply sitting still and holding their head up against gravity is not enough for them to feel secure about what their body is doing. They need more and will move until they arrive at that point of optimum arousal. In order to get this, they may rock in their seat, shake their leg, or constantly squirm in their seat. I saw a great dramatization of this in which an elementary aged boy is rocking back and forth in his chair saying, "I can focus. I can focus. I can focus." In the background you hear the teacher tell him to sit still in his chair. He listens, but once he is sitting still he is saying, "I can't focus. I can't focus. I can't focus." He needed the movement and input to his vestibular system in order to reach an optimum level of arousal so he could focus on what the teacher was saying and on his school work. With my own son, I never ask him to sit still and look me in the eye when I am trying to talk to him or get my point across. He can listen and focus better when he is moving or fidgeting with something. I allow him to move while I am talking to him, but I always ask for him to repeat what I just said. Sure enough, he always can. If I made him sit still while I spoke to him, I guarantee you that he wouldn't hear a word because he does not focus best in this state.

- **Seek out intense movement** – Do your children love to spin, jump, and move fast? Does it seem like they are not having fun unless they are moving quickly? Some children could swing for days or spin for hours and never get dizzy or ride amusement park rides all day and not get sick. These kids may have a hard time when it comes to activities that require them to slow down because they crave what Doreit Bailer *(A Secret Revealed, 2011)* calls "fun fast faster." They will find ways to do things faster and typically turn a safe activity into a dangerous one.
- **Always run to their destination** – Do your children seem to only have one speed and that is fast? They have to run, hop, jump, etc. to get to where they are going and walking just won't get the job done. They need the fast and more intense movement that running provides their vestibular systems. My son was like this. I knew as soon as he was awake because I could hear his feet running down the hallway. As soon as his feet hit the floor in the morning, he ran. It seemed it was his only mode of transportation.
- **Dare-devil** – Do your children seem to have "no fears" or to be "thrill seekers"? Some children need intense movement. Just jumping off the ground is not enough. They need to jump from higher surfaces, climb higher, swing faster, and can make any activity seem a little more dangerous.

Signs of low muscle tone or poor coordination

- **Floppy limbs** – Could you tie your children's arms behind their backs like wet noodles and not hurt them? It isn't caused by a lack of strength. Instead it is the result of low muscle tone. This condition is the result of the vestibular system's connection with the vestibulo-spinal reflex which helps to stabilize our posture and maintain muscle control. When the vestibular system is not functioning correctly, muscle tone will be affected causing what is called *hypotonia,* or decreased muscle tone. These children will appear floppy or may sometimes seem as though they are double jointed. Hypotonicity can lead to problems with postural control, difficulties with gross and fine motor skills, and oral motor coordination deficits. The movement of our arms, legs, and head depends on good postural control. When children have low muscle tone, they lack the postural control needed for stability off which their extremities and head work.

- **Fine motor and gross motor deficits** – Do your children have difficulty using tools such as pencils, scissors, and silverware or learning to ride a bike, catch and throw a ball, do jumping jacks, etc.? The muscle tone we just talked about can play an important role with these skills. Muscle tone is needed for postural or trunk control and stability, and postural and trunk stability are needed for sufficient use of our limbs. If children have low muscle tone and poor postural stability, they will have difficulty with coordinated movements. Another reason for this is that the vestibular system plays a part in bilateral coordination or learning to use the two sides of our bodies together in a coordinated manner, as well as in our eye-hand and eye-foot coordination. When there is a problem with these skills, coordinated movements will suffer.
- **"W" sitting** – Do your children seem to be unable to or avoid sitting "criss-cross applesauce"? "W" sitting is when children sit on the floor with their knees bent and lower leg out to the side of their upper leg (as opposed to crossed in front when sitting criss-cross applesauce.) Children with low muscle tone will prefer to sit this way because it gives them a wider base of support for increased stability.
- **Ambidextrous** – Does it seem as though your children have never established a dominant hand even after the age of 4 or 5? Does it seem as though one hand does not seem more skilled than the other? As I mentioned earlier, the vestibular system places a role in bilateral coordination, as well as helping a child develop a side (or a hand) that is more skilled than the other.
- **Fatigues easily** – Do your children seem to lose their steam more quickly than their peers? With decreased muscle tone and postural control, it is easy to understand why these children would fatigue more easily. Everything they do requires a lot more effort because they are working off of an unstable base.

THE VESTIBULAR (VES-TIB-U-LAR) SYSTEM

Over-sensitive to vestibular input

- **Seem fearful of movement** – Do your children seem to be uncomfortable with changes in movement and having their feet leave the ground? Activities that can invoke this fear may be jumping, swinging, sliding, balancing, climbing, learning to ride a bike, going on an elevator or escalator, walking up or down stairs, leaning back for an activity such as washing their hair in the sink, being tipped upside down, or riding in a car.
- **Get motion sick easily** – Do your children get nauseated or dizzy easily in response to movement such as spinning or riding in a car? An oversensitivity to movement can cause this physiological reaction.
- **Prefer sedentary activities** – Are your children "couch potatoes" or "mouse potatoes" (who could sit and play video games all day long)? Children who are oversensitive to vestibular input and the way it makes them feel may choose not to move much at all. They may avoid activities that require their feet to leave the ground or challenges to their balance.
- **Appear clumsy** – Do your children seem to lose their balance easily or fall frequently? Do they seem to struggle with hand-eye or foot-eye coordination? The vestibular system plays a large role in our balance and our visual system. This can lead to difficulty with, or a fear of, tasks that require balance such as learning to ride a bike, walking on a curb or balance beam, or balancing or hopping on one foot. Oftentimes, if you ask these children to balance on one foot with their eyes closed, they will have even greater problems because now they have to rely more heavily on their vestibular system. These children may also have difficulty catching a ball, kicking a rolling ball, buttoning buttons, cutting with scissors, or just seem very uncoordinated in the way that they use their bodies.

You might have noticed that some of the signs of proprioceptive deficits and vestibular deficits look similar. You are right. These two systems work very closely together as the information is gathered through the movement of our heads *and* bodies. As I mentioned in chapter 2, these two systems help children to know where they are. These systems come together to form our **kinesthetic awareness** which combines our sense of movement with our sense of position of our body.

Think of riding a bike—you need a great sense of balance as well as a great sense of what your legs are doing as you pedal (since, hopefully, you are looking up at where you are going and not at your feet). This is kinesthetics at its finest, and it takes the proprioceptive and vestibular systems (along with tactile and visual systems) working hand in hand to make this activity successful.

> Children who are constantly on the go and can't sit still may be SEEKING OUT proprioceptive or vestibular input or both.

Children who are constantly on the go and can't sit still may be seeking out proprioceptive or vestibular input or both. The good news is though, that using activities to build both their proprioceptive and vestibular foundations will work and many activities we do (such as jumping, climbing, running, balancing, etc.) provide children with both types of input at the same time.

What is important for you to realize is that the reason the children can't sit still is not that they are bad or defiant kids; instead, they don't feel secure until they move. As stated by Athena Oden in *Ready Bodies Learning Minds (2006)*, "Once a child learns to move against gravity effectively, only then will he be able to develop control and learn to maintain stillness."

REMEMBER: You have to LEARN TO MOVE and MOVE TO LEARN!

Refer to chapter 24 for a list of activities that you can do with your children to help build their vestibular system.

CHAPTER 14

THE TACTILE (TAC-TILE) SYSTEM

The tactile system is our largest sensory system. This system processes information regarding touch, temperature, texture, vibration, and pain. You may want to take a minute to go back to chapter 2 and review this system and its two subsystems, the discriminative and protective systems. The discriminative subsystem gives us the information regarding the qualities of a tactile stimulus such as whether it is hot or cold, soft or hard, gives us deep or light pressure, bumpy or smooth, painful or pleasant, etc. The protective subsystem is the one that puts us on high alert or makes us respond quickly and emotionally to a tactile stimulus that is or that we perceive as being harmful (such as a bug crawling on our leg or when we accidentally touch a hot stove).

I also mentioned in chapter 2 that the tactile system plays an important role in our behavior. So why is this? In that chapter, I talked about this system's connection with our "fight, flight, or fright" system (or our sympathetic nervous system). When there is faulty functioning of either the protective or discriminative system, children may interpret ordinary touch as noxious, threatening, or harmful, setting their "fight, flight, or fright" system into high gear. When this happens, we may see behaviors that concern us—tantrums, screaming, hitting, aggression, or avoidance just to name a few. Without knowledge of *why* they are acting this way, their behaviors may be interpreted as defiant, problematic, or simply bad.

Let me give you an example here. Think about children standing in line to go out to recess or walk down to the cafeteria. The expectation is that they can be still, quiet, and follow in line behind the person in front of them without causing any problems. Not too much to ask, right? Well, if you have children standing in that line who have tactile dysfunction or sensitivity, it just might completely overwhelm them. Think of all the opportunities for those children to accidentally receive tactile input from the other children near them. Other children may accidentally brush up against them or rub them with their jacket, shirt sleeve, or backpack if they stand too close. This accidental brushing or light touch may cause the children to kick into "fight, flight, or fright" mode. Instead of just processing the characteristics of this touch, such as soft, light, cold, etc. (discriminatory system), your children may process it as noxious and potentially harmful; thus their protective system kicks in. For some children, it may be standing in line or any other crowded situation that causes this. For other children, it may be the feeling of their clothes against their skin, certain textures that they eat, or getting their hands or feet dirty that cause them to kick into "fight, flight, or fright" mode.

Put yourself in your children's shoes for a minute and think about all of the situations they go through during the school day where they are exposed to touch from objects or people that are outside of their control. On the school bus, children sit too close and brush up against you or someone walking to their seat brushes against you with their body or backpack. The teacher may have a fun new activity to do that day that requires touching or manipulating some totally new texture. The kids on the playground want to play freeze tag and are constantly touching in order to tag you. Mom packs something new in your lunchbox or the cafeteria is serving something that has an unfamiliar taste and texture. During circle time, you have to sit on a soft carpet that tickles your legs and Sally next to you always sits too close and touches your knee with hers as she sits criss-cross applesauce. You get off of the school bus, probably at the end of your rope from all of this, and now mom or dad wants to take you to get your haircut. Are you serious? After all of this, "I now have to let a total stranger touch my head with a sharp object in his/her hand or electric clippers buzzing right in my ear?"

Do you get it now? When your tactile system is working perfectly, these situations don't even faze you. You don't think twice about someone brushing up against you or touching something different or novel to you. However, when there is immaturity, sensitivity, modulation problems, or dysfunction in children's tactile systems, this school day may be so overwhelming to them and they may act accordingly. Instead of registering the discriminatory qualities of each of these touches, the children are in "fight, flight, or fright" mode because their protective system is beating out the discriminative system.

Let me give you a few more examples of "fight, flight, or fright" behaviors that I have seen from children who have difficulty modulating tactile input:
- I have a friend who strongly encouraged her son to eat mashed potatoes with the family at dinner. He was very hesitant, but after some strong negotiating, he tried them. He then proceeded to run away from the table and up to his room crying. The texture of the mashed potatoes caused his sensory cup to overflow and put him in to "flight" mode.

- A girl named Brittany, with whom I worked in the clinic, did not like to be touched. Many of the younger kids don't mind holding my hand when transitioning from the lobby to the gym or from one activity to another. Brittany, however, wanted nothing to do with that. I needed to find a way to help her transition because she loved to take off running, so instead of holding her hand, I held on to one end of a swimming pool noodle and she held onto the other end. She was completely fine and felt safe with that. After some time working with her, she was willing to hold my hand but it took a few months of building her sensory foundation to get there.
- Another little girl with whom I worked, Meagan, got asked to leave kindergarten after two days. Meagan seemed as though she was a real bully. She would punch other kids for what seemed to be no reason at all. At least, what seemed like no reason at all. What was actually happening was that she was being touched, brushed up against, etc., and her system couldn't take it. Meagan acted out in the way that her nervous system was telling her to act, as she perceived these actions as potentially dangerous. She "fought."

For every one of these "fight, flight, or fright" children, there is a child who has to touch *everything*. These are the children who have to come into the clinic and touch everything they see before they are able to get to work. They are the ones who touch everything they see in the store or who have you fiddle with mom's bracelet, necklace, or shirt while talking to them. This is my son who is constantly holding on to his shirt just below the collar (It's as though it was his security blanket.) and my daughter who is obsessed with soft, plush stuffed animals. These kids need touch and need more of it. They *need* this extra input in order to fill their tactile cup to the level it needs to be for optimum level of arousal. I could ask my son all day long to let go of his shirt, but he would just end up trading that habit for another tactile habit. What he is showing me is that he needs to touch something, that he is craving more tactile input.

Like the other sensory systems, the tactile system can be one where children can have difficulty modulating input and may be over or under-sensitive. Some children are under-sensitive and need more tactile input in order to reach an optimum level of arousal; so they will seek it out. Other children are tactilely defensive, or hypersensitive to touch input and will let you know through the way they act in response to touch or the things they avoid. Let me give you a brief list of some of the behaviors you may see in children who have a hunger for more tactile input or who are defensive toward it.

Under-sensitive to tactile input

- **Touch everything or everyone** – These children may seek out the touch of a soft blanket or objects that provide stronger tactile input (such as spikey, bumpy, or rough objects). They may seem as if they are always touching you, whether they are rubbing your clothes, twirling your necklace, holding on to your leg, or just sitting or standing close enough to you to be touching you at all times. I have a balance cushion in the clinic that I have children stand on. It has a smooth side and a side with lots of little rubbery spikes. Children who seek out extra tactile input will always prefer to stand on the side with the spikes while the defensive kids will refuse that side opting for the smooth side. My daughter LOVES stuffed animals and is very attached to some of the softer ones. Each time she sees them, it's as though she just saw her long lost best friend. She loves to rub them against her face and feel the softness against her bare skin. A funny observation that I have made is that the children I know who crave tactile input seem to love dogs. Think about all of the tactile input children receive from petting a dog.
- **Prefer messy play** – These children may seem to gravitate toward activities that will get their hands dirty. They may also not seem to notice when they have food on their face or have dirty hands.
- **Seem unaware of cuts, scrapes, bruises, or other injuries** – These children may not respond to a minor injury that may bother the rest of us. This is because the injury was not great enough to register with them that it occurred.
- **Seem to cause injury to themselves** – These children may bang their head, pinch themselves, bite their nails, etc. just to give themselves the extra tactile input that they need.
- **Frequently mouths object** – I mentioned this in the proprioceptive chapter; however, it can also fall under the tactile category. Children may excessively put things in their mouth for the tactile input that they get through exploring the object

through their mouth and may use their mouths to learn about the tactile qualities of an object. When children mouth objects for proprioceptive input, they will generally chew and bite on the object using the heavy work muscles of the mouth to do so.

Over-sensitive to tactile input

- **Seem anxious or fearful of light touch** – These are the children that move their arms away when you go to touch them. They may also become over-aroused or anxious when the teacher goes to touch them to redirect them or give them hand over hand assistance with a project or task. They may also avoid or get distressed by situations in which they will have to stand in a line or other crowded situations where they may be touched.
- **Doesn't like having hair combed or cut, nails trimmed, teeth brushed, or face washed** – Think about it. If children are fearful of being touched and now you are coming at them with a foreign, textured, or sharp object, you can imagine what this will do to them (especially if it is being done by someone the children don't know or haven't learned to trust).
- **Resists being hugged or cuddled** – This can be by strangers or by loved ones. For children to have someone coming at them, wanting to touch them in an unpredictable way, can be very stressful to children who don't like to be touched.
- **Avoids messy play and getting their hands dirty** – These children will not want to finger paint, glue, or play in the mud. They may feel the need to wash their hands as soon as they feel them get a little dirty. I use foam soap a lot in the clinic when teaching handwriting. Most kids love to smear it all around the cookie sheet and will even rub the soap all over their arms and face. Not the kids who don't like touch. Those kids refuse to touch the soap and prefer to use a paintbrush for the activity instead so they don't have to experience the feel of it on their hands.
- **Does not like tags or the feeling of certain clothes on them** – If you are sensitive to touch, the constant feeling of your clothes on your body will bother you. For most of us, we get used to the feeling of our clothes against our bodies very quickly, and we

don't give it a second thought throughout our day. Not so with children who are "defensive." These children may have a hard time accommodating to the feeling of the clothes and may also be very particular about the seams on their socks being in just the right place or be very particular about wearing short vs long sleeves or pants vs shorts.

- **Be a picky eater** – Children are not always picky eaters because they don't like the taste of a certain food. Often times, they don't like the texture of a certain food and the tactile input that they get from it. You may find that the food they dislike has the same tactile qualities (for example, crunchy, mushy, mealy, or slimy). You may also find that the foods that they do like, all have the same tactile qualities.
- **Tiptoe walking** – I talked about this one in Chapter 12 when I discussed a possible explanation for tiptoe walking as children being under-responsive to proprioceptive input. A second explanation for tiptoe walking is a tactile over-responsiveness. In this case, you may tend to notice this more when children are barefoot because the tactile input they get through the soles of their feet touching the ground (or even grass or sand) becomes too much for them.
- **Avoids showering or gets distressed by rain drops or water falling on them** – Water coming down on them, especially in a way that the children can't control, provides touch input to them that can cause fear and anxiety and, because of this, they will avoid it.
- **Dislikes walking or sitting in sand or on grass** – These can be a very noxious feeling to children who are defensive.
- **Overreacts to minor cuts or scrapes** – To them, these injuries that seem minor to us are much more painful and threatening. Their brains may not be registering that this is a minor cut, but instead, are telling them that this is a terribly painful injury.

Poor tactile discrimination

Tactile Discrimination: Distinguishing between the characteristics of the sensory input (hot/cold, sharp/dull, smooth/rough, etc).

- **Difficulty with fine motor tasks** – This can include things such as buttoning, zipping, tying shoes, etc. When children have a hard time making sense of the tactile qualities of an object, they will have a hard time formulating a motor plan for what to do with those objects.
- **Difficulty manipulating tools (or objects they hold in their hand)** – This can include using scissors, silverware, crayons, a pencil, a paintbrush, etc. As mentioned above, if children do not perceive the feel of an object appropriately so that they are able to discriminate between the qualities of it: hard/soft, big/little, soft/rough, etc., they will have a hard time figuring out how to manipulate it.
- **May have a hard time identifying objects by feel alone** – If children have a hard time discriminating between the tactile qualities of an object, they will not be able to locate an object based on feel alone and will need to use vision. This will make it hard for them to reach in to a backpack and pull out a particular object without seeing it or to reach in to a box and pick out a crayon vs. a pencil without seeing it.

Refer to chapter 25 for activities that you can do with your child to help build their tactile system.

CHAPTER 15

SENSORY PROCESSING DISORDER

Now that we have talked about the sensory foundation and what it looks like when it is immature or when there is a dysfunction (particularly in the near senses), I want to take some time to explain some of the diagnoses that involve dysfunction with the sensory system. By doing so, I want you to understand the importance of working with your children (with the direction of a therapist) to build their sensory foundation in order to help them gain the skills needed for emotional and behavioral regulation and motor performance.

The first diagnosis I want to explain is Sensory Processing Disorder (SPD), formerly known as "sensory integration dysfunction." This is the diagnosis that is given to children when their sensory processing problems cause interference in their daily functioning. SPD exists when the sensory input received doesn't get organized into appropriate responses. Sensory information (such as that regarding movement, touch, sound, sight) is sensed but misinterpreted. When this information is misinterpreted, children will then experience the world around them differently.

Dr. Jean Ayres (1979) compares this condition to a neurological "traffic jam" where certain parts of the brain are blocked from receiving the information it needs to interpret sensory information correctly. She says that the brain must organize all of the incoming sensations in order to move and learn and behave normally. She states that, "the brain locates, sorts, and orders sensations—somewhat like a traffic policeman directing moving cars. When sensations flow in a well-integrated manner, the brain can use those sensations to form perceptions, behaviors, and learning. When the flow of sensations is disorganized, life can be like a rush-hour traffic jam."

Children with SPD have difficulty processing the information they receive through their senses which, in turn, makes functioning in everyday life challenging. These children may feel bombarded and overwhelmed by what seem like ordinary sensations. If untreated, SPD may result in motor performance problems, behavioral problems, avoidance of certain sensory experiences, aggression, problems with socialization, coordination deficits, anxiety, depression, learning challenges, trouble focusing, a troubled self-esteem, and many other issues.

SPD has started to become a household name over the last few years with the number of children affected on the rise. One study (Ahn, Miller, Milberger, McIntosh, 2004) shows that at least 1 in 20 children's daily lives is affected by SPD. We know that SPD is on the rise, but the good news is that more and more research and information are becoming available.

I am not going to go into too much detail on all of the categories of dysfunction that fall under SPD for the purposes of this book, but I do want to address Sensory Modulation Disorder (a category or pattern of SPD) and its subtypes. The reason for this being that this is where I find many children are struggling either mildly or more severely. I want you to have a clear picture of Sensory Modulation Disorder and its subtypes and their relationship to the sensory foundation. This will then help you to understand what you need to be looking for in these children and what you can do to help them.

Sensory modulation refers to our ability to regulate our responses in a way that is proportional to the sensory stimulation we receive. Our brains have filters which allow us to take in the "just right" amount of sensory information needed to function but kick out extraneous information in order to keep us from being bombarded by sensory input. These filters also help to regulate the amount and intensity of sensory information that the brain processes.

In children with Sensory Modulation Disorder (called SMD) there is a problem with these filters and the way the nervous system

> SENSORY MODULATION refers to our ability to regulate our responses in a way that is proportional to the sensory stimulation we receive.

adjusts to, regulates, limits, or enhances incoming sensory input. Modulation should take place automatically; therefore, allowing children to maintain an optimum level of arousal. However, in children with SMD this is not the case. To a child with SMD, sensory stimuli may seem as if it is coming through like someone screaming in a megaphone or someone whispering so quietly you can barely hear them - and sometimes there is no in-between.

Sensory modulation dysfunction is on a continuum, from children who will try to avoid nearly all stimulation to children who will seek out as much stimulation as they can. Many children will actually do a combination of both depending on their arousal level. An arousal level can vary throughout the day since modulation occurs every second of every day as children receive input to at least one of their senses at all times. This can make life with children with SPD very unpredictable!

I briefly explained sensory over and under-sensitivities in chapter 9. I compared these two states to cups, sensory cups as I like to call them. Remember that children's sensory cups need to be at the "just right" level so they don't spill over, yet are full enough to quench their thirst. That "just right" amount of liquid can be associated with helping them to reach and maintain that optimum level of arousal. I want to talk more about these sensory cups as they relate to SMD and children with sensory under responsiveness and sensory over responsiveness. These classifications become important when we talk about SMD because this will help you to understand your children's behaviors so that you can then know what to do to help them.

Sensory under responsiveness

Children with sensory under responsiveness (SUR) have a cup that takes a lot to fill it up (It may seem more like a big pitcher than a cup). Remember that only when the cup is filled to an optimum level that children will be able to work efficiently. Otherwise, they will be left still thirsty from not enough liquid to satisfy them. These children are still thirsty because they haven't had enough and need more. They may need an enormous amount of liquid to fill their cup or need constant refueling to keep the cup at an optimum level. If their cup does not reach a high enough level, their level of arousal will suffer, and they will have difficulty engaging or participating in activities in a meaningful way. These children may need stimulation that lasts longer and that is of greater intensity and will need quick bursts of stimuli to fill their cup and get to their optimum level of arousal.

These children can vary in their response to their under responsiveness. According to Bailer and Miller (2011), children with SUR seem to keep their thoughts and feelings inside and tend to get lost in a fantasy world that can seem a lot like autism. They may even seem numb. When you can get their sensory cup filled to the level it needs to be, however, they often come to life and are able to be productive. These children may have difficulty following directions or responding to having their name called. They may seem withdrawn or under aroused. They may not notice certain smells or strong tastes. They may have low muscle tone because of how much input it takes to reach their threshold, and therefore, the neurological connection to the muscles is weak.

Children with SUR can also seem hyperactive as they may bounce from one thing to another and seek out all kinds of movement experiences in order to fill their cup. These children need movement and more sensory input to get their huge cup filled to the point at which they are at their optimum level of arousal. Telling them to sit still over and over will be a pointless endeavor; they can't. Well, they can; however, they won't be able to focus when sitting still because their cup isn't filled. Let them move and they will increase their ability to focus.

Robbie's Story

Robbie is a 10-year-old boy with SUR. Robbie's parents have been told by his teachers that he has ADHD. He can't sit still in class and focus; he is always fidgeting. He also has a hard time with peer interactions, has poor self-esteem, has few friends, and often plays by himself at recess. Robbie never seems to hear his name being called, is withdrawn, and cannot identify his or other's emotions very well. He also has a weak trunk and arms, struggles with fine motor skills, touches everything he sees, and has a mild speech delay. His parent's biggest concern at this point is his lack of emotional regulation, self-control, and self-esteem. He just doesn't know how to handle himself in social situations. They are actually curious at this point if he falls somewhere on the autism spectrum.

When you start to get to the root Robbie's problem, you realize that many of the behaviors and problems he has are caused by SUR. He has an auditory under responsiveness (doesn't hear his name being called). He has a vestibular under responsiveness (poor muscle control and weakness and a need to constantly fidget). Robbie has a tactile under responsiveness (constantly touching EVERYTHING). He can't sit still in class and is tuned out because his cup is not full. Robbie's sensory foundation is suffering; therefore, his motor performance and emotional and behavioral regulation are suffering as well.

Robbie is not reaching his optimum level of arousal because he has a hard time adjusting to and regulating (modulating) the sensory input he is receiving. He lives in a state of under arousal. That is no way to get through your day successfully. I think if I had to go through life feeling under aroused like I do on a Monday morning that it would be tough! Robbie just doesn't have a clear understanding of what is going on within his own body because of this; so we really can't expect him to understand others or what they are feeling if he doesn't even understand what is going on inside of him. This under arousal leads to his withdrawn behavior and trouble with peer relationships, and this is not good because he is at an age where friendships form the basis of self-esteem.

Once Robbie's parents are able to gain a clear understanding of *why* he is behaving the way he is and *why* he is having struggles, they can start to identify what it is that he really needs at a given moment and provide it for him. This includes giving intense and quick bursts of sensory input. It is so important for him to get the sensory input that will help him reach his threshold and fill his cup so he can reach his optimal level of arousal. This process, in turn, will help him build his sensory foundation and make those foundational levels of building blocks strong and sturdy so that his emotional and behavioral regulation and motor performance will then improve.

Jake's Story

Jake is a third grader who came to me for help with his handwriting. He originally came to my house for private tutoring sessions. At the time in which Jake's parents contacted me, they were getting very frustrated. He had just started on ADD medication but was struggling in school with focusing, getting his work done, and with his handwriting. He had been placed into the gifted and talented program at school but was falling behind. They were having a hard time getting the school to give him any extra assistance or accommodations, and they felt like they were spinning their wheels and beating their heads up against a brick wall.

It didn't take me long to see that Jake had sensory processing problems, and specifically, sensory modulation deficits. He had a very hard time sitting still in his chair to work on his handwriting. He touched everything around him, squirmed in his chair, and had a very short attention span. I also started to notice that he had a weak trunk and poor postural stability as he had a hard time writing on the chalkboard having to brace himself with one arm and stick his tongue out in an attempt to compensate for his weak trunk. I started to notice something else that was interesting about Jake; he would frequently ask me to slow down when we were doing our work.

I quickly kicked out of handwriting tutor mode and into OT mode so I could get him to focus. Since he could not sit still and had to fidget, touch things, and squirm, I realized that his cup was not full and he was trying to fill it. I started giving him opportunities to fill his cup throughout our sessions. We would work for five minutes then exercise for a few minutes then work for five minutes, exercise, etc. I would have him jump on my indoor trampoline, punch the punching bag, spin on my spin board, do the wheelbarrow down the hall, or stand on the balance board while tossing the medicine ball. I was trying to give him lots of proprioceptive input (and some vestibular input, as well) while we worked. Instead of sitting in a chair to work on his writing, I had him lie down on the floor on his stomach prop on his elbows; therefore, increasing the amount of proprioceptive input he got while writing. This worked like a charm. We started having great sessions. I filled his cup so he could focus and repeatedly gave him refills to help maintain his engagement in his work.

What I realized with Jake was that he was slow to process auditory information, as well. That is why he repeatedly asked me to slow down. That is also why he was falling behind in his work at school. The teacher in the gifted program would give verbal instructions and then let the kids do their work accordingly. Jake wasn't getting it. He wasn't understanding from just the verbal instructions and was too shy or embarrassed to speak up. I brought everything to his parents' attention that I had noticed so they could take the information back to his school and seek out outpatient Occupational Therapy in a clinic setting.

If you have children who do not seem to respond to sensory input, who seem withdrawn, or who appear to seek out more intense sensory input, it is not necessarily a behavior problem, bad parenting, or ADHD. It may be the result of their sensory system that is just not giving them enough stimulation to fill their cup to the level needed for optimum arousal; they may need so much more and may be in search of it. They may need more intense sensory input to get their engine running. Contact your physician and inquire about Occupational Therapy if you suspect your child has SUR. You can also look for some ideas on how to help them by working sensory input in to their day. Please reference chapter 26 for an extensive list of ideas.

Sensory over responsiveness

Sensory over responsiveness (called SOR) is the term we use to describe it when children's cups get filled very quickly. This happens because they have a low threshold for certain sensory inputs. It doesn't take much sensory stimuli to get their cup to overflowing, and they may become too excited or too over-aroused to participate meaningfully in an activity. In children with SOR, evidence suggests that the functioning of the sympathetic nervous system (the "fight, flight, or fright" system) differs significantly from that of "typically developing" children. Their "fight, flight, or fright" system responds more frequently and with greater magnitude and often does not habituate to (or get accustomed to) sensory input.

SOR children may avoid certain objects or situations or show aversions or fears because they know that certain stimuli will take them to that state of overflow quickly. They may be in a constant state of high alert. When that cup overflows, you will often see emotional or behavioral reactions which may seem out of proportion to the stimuli that were received. This reaction occurs because the "fight, flight, or fright" aspect of their nervous system takes over in response to the stimuli. When children feel bombarded or overwhelmed by sensory stimuli, their nervous systems may process this as a threat and let the autonomic nervous system take over. With SOR, children often have trouble screening out extraneous stimuli. They may attend to every little noise they hear, be bothered by the feeling of the clothes on their skin, or become overwhelmed by too much visual stimuli in the classroom making it hard for them to attend visually to the work on their desk.

I am going to use myself as an example here. For me, a trip to the local indoor bounce house facility or pizza place with the singing animals on stage will fill my cup to a point of overflow very quickly. All of the visual and auditory stimuli put me in meltdown mode. It does not take much noise to fill my cup. I do not enjoy movie theaters for that reason, and my poor husband will never get to put surround sound in our house because I am constantly requesting that the TV gets turned down. When my kids have friends over, they love to ride their indoor riding toys around and around on a path they have figured out on the hardwoods through the kitchen, family room, foyer, and dining room (and scream really loud while they do it). They are usually also yelling, "Mrs. Cindy, Mrs. Cindy, Mrs. Cindy" over and over with different requests (and perhaps a little whining may also occur). I handle it, though, and can maintain my composure for a period of time. However, it only takes one tiny thing to happen after the riding toys have been put away for me to blow a fuse and lose my cool. This happens because my auditory cup is just at the brink of overflowing and one other little thing will quickly take it to an overflow state. The same thing happens in the car on the way home from the bounce house facility of pizza place with video games and singing animals. My kids start yelling for one reason or another in the car and, boom, I lose my cool. My cup is sitting on the brink of overflow and the added yelling pushes me over the top.

An example of this kind of response is that of children who are afraid to swing or slide because to do so will make their vestibular cup fill too quickly. Still other examples are those of children who avoid certain foods or textures because they fill their tactile cup too quickly, or children who appear clumsy or who are fearful of difficult learning situations such as riding a bike. I mentioned in chapter 14 the story about a friend of mine who really wanted her son to try mashed potatoes at dinner. She just knew he would like them and the old "you have to just try one bite" strategy kicked in. Well, he tried a bite after much encouragement and ran off to his room screaming, "Why?" because his brain perceived the texture of those potatoes as a noxious stimulus, and it activated his "fight, flight, or fright" system. He's a great kid, this stimulus was just too much for him.

Hope's Story

Hope is a nine-year-old girl brought in to me by her mother, initially for handwriting problems. Hope is another example of a child whose struggle with a skill at the top of the building blocks of learning (poor handwriting) was something her mother could see and for which she knew she could get help. Hope is also another example of a child who, when we did some investigating, is struggling with not having an adequate foundation of her building blocks of learning which is leading to her struggles with her motor skills. What I discovered after spending some time with her and talking to her mom was that she had a lot of sensory over responsiveness and a great deal of fear because of this.

Hope's mother was very concerned over the number of fears that she had. Hope has a five-year-old sister whom she would send in ahead of her to check out the new situation or whom she would have try new things first, and then Hope would decide if she wanted to try it based on her sister's feedback. Hope was very resistant to trying anything new and needed a great deal of reassurance before attempting to use any of the equipment in the clinic. Hope did not like to be in crowds or in situations where she had to stand in close proximity to other people for fear of being touched by them. She did not like having her hair brushed or cut or having her nails cut. She also did not like getting her hands dirty or participating in "messy play." Hope preferred sedentary activities and was VERY cautious. She had difficulty with gross motor skills such as catching a ball. She was afraid of heights, afraid of falling, and afraid of activities that required her feet to leave the ground.

Hope also had a lot of auditory over responsiveness and found it quite hard to concentrate or focus if there were any auditory distractions around. She was the kind of child who disliked loud noises and refused to go to a movie theater because of this. Hope was the kind of child who noticed everything going on around her and could not tune out any visual or auditory stimulus.

Another behavior that Hope exhibited that was especially frustrating to her mother was her "OCD-like tendencies." Hope had to have everything in a certain place and did not handle it well when things were out of place. When she and I worked together in the clinic, she spent a lot of time fixing the components of the activity or the game we were playing. Everything had to be just right before we got started.

Because of all of Hope's hypersensitivities to sensory input, she tried at all costs to avoid situations in which she would be exposed to these types of stimuli. You can only imagine then, what happens to a child's foundation (the sensory building block) when they avoid interacting with their environment in ways that will help to build their foundation . . . it becomes a vicious cycle. Their foundation is going to suffer and not be nearly as strong as it needs to be in order to support the rest of the building blocks. As a result of a faulty foundation, Hope struggled in the areas of emotional and behavioral regulation and motor performance. Her fears and avoidance of things and situations were starting to interfere with her daily performance, and her motor skills (such as handwriting, catching a ball, and activities such as monkey bars that required upper body strength) were suffering. Her need for things to be exactly right before starting a game or for every toy to be in its place was also becoming a big concern. Like many children with SOR, Hope liked to have things just right and didn't like changes. Any little change, or having to deal with something that isn't just right, can throw children with SOR's sensory systems into overload as it tries to figure out how to deal with the lack of predictability or the change.

The goal with Hope was to first educate her mom on *why* she reacted the way she did to certain situations (situations that would cause her sensory system to go into "fight, flight, or fright") and *why* she was struggling in the motor performance areas. Next, it was important for Hope and her mom to have a bag of tricks, a plethora of activities to use at home and in the environment to help her to self-regulate in fear evoking situations and to help build her sensory foundation. Once we could build her sensory foundation, we would then start to see an improvement in the areas of emotional and behavioral regulation and motor performance. In the clinic, my goal was to expose Hope to as much vestibular, proprioceptive, and tactile input as possible but to do it in a way that did not feel threatening to her and often requiring us to build up or build on previous experiences to increase the challenge. We started slowly but built up to doing a great deal of spinning, swinging, jumping, rolling, riding on the scooter board, playing in the rice bowl, and with foam soap. We used a lot of deep pressure, when needed, to give calming and organizing input so she was able to tolerate these vestibular and proprioceptive challenges. Another goal for Hope was to increase her upper body and trunk strength. We did this through providing vestibular and proprioceptive input and through using positions in which she had to bear weight though her arms (wheelbarrowing, crab walking, holding a plank position, doing puzzles or playing games on the floor on all fours, and holding on while swinging from a trapeze or monkey bar). We did address her handwriting needs, but only after we used this sensory input to get her brain neurologically ready to learn.

Once we did all of this, Hope was able to become more confident about her body and what it was capable of, her sensory foundation was broadened, and neuroplastic changes to her brain were made (I will talk about this in greater detail in chapter 20). Because of this, she was better able to tolerate sensory input (instead of avoiding it), her fears decreased, and her motor skills improved.

I will talk about this more in chapter 18, but I want to point out here that many children with SMD, and specifically SOR, have fears and anxiety. Hope's story is a good example of this. One of the reasons why children with SOR may have fears and anxiety is that anything new that may feel, smell, sound, or look different or any novel situation that will provide unpredictable sensory stimulation can be very challenging for them. They just don't know what sensory stimulus they are going to receive, and this can be very scary for them and lead them to respond or behave in a way that is alarming to us, at least until we understand *why* they are acting as they are and *how* we can help them.

I mentioned earlier that because we are receiving some sort of sensory input at all times, we have to modulate that input every second of the day (even though most of us don't have to ever even think about it). Because of this, over and under responsiveness can vary from day-to-day and can vary from one context to another. This means that children can be over responsive to, let's say, tactile input one day or in one setting and under responsive the next day or in a different environment. Children may also be over responsive in regards to one of their senses and under responsive in regards to another. If you did the math on it, there are over 29,000,000 different combinations of sensory challenges that children can face. An example of this may be children who are over responsive to loud noises and food textures. This means that exposure to loud, unexpected noise or experiencing a new food texture will cause them to exhibit a breakdown in the emotional/behavioral regulation performance area and reach a point of overarousal. They may have a tantrum or meltdown, act aggressively (such as biting or hitting), or begin to avoid any situations in which the threat of experiencing that sensory stimulus may occur. Those same children may be under responsive to vestibular and/or proprioceptive input and have a hard time sitting still exhibiting the need to fidget or move constantly. These children need more movement input to fill that cup to register that something is happening and get to their optimum level of arousal. Therefore, they must move more to get that input.

If you look for cues, you will be able to put the pieces of the puzzle together in order to give your children more of what they need or help them work through the areas where they need less. When you see your children avoid or react negatively to an object, activity, or situation and you can figure out what that object, activity, or situation is doing to their sensory system that is causing them to act a certain way, you can start to figure out what to do to help them. Then, what you can do is provide appropriate activities that will give them what they need to help them avoid the negative response or avoidance, and you can do it frequently. This will, in turn, help them to reach and maintain an optimum level of arousal. When you understand *why* they are behaving as they are, you may be more understanding of what they are doing and be better equipped to help them.

Refer to chapter 27 for a list of activities that you can do with your child who exhibits signs of SOR.

CHAPTER 16

ADD/ADHD AND THE SENSORY SYSTEM

Now that I have explained an immature sensory system, sensory integration, and you know more about what Sensory Processing Disorder (specifically Sensory Modulation Disorder) looks like, we need to talk about ADD and ADHD and their link with the sensory system and the sensory foundation. There are a lot of similar behaviors seen in children who have been diagnosed with ADD or ADHD and kids with immature sensory systems or Sensory Processing Disorder (SPD). As reported by Dr. Lucy Jane Miller (one of the top researchers in sensory integration/sensory processing disorders) in an article in Parents Magazine in June 2000, "more than half of children suspected to have ADHD actually had sensory integration dysfunction or BOTH conditions." Children with ADD/ADHD can have a wide variety of ways in which they process sensory information, and studies show, specifically, that they tend to be more sensitive to sensory stimuli than children without ADD or ADHD.

It can be hard to distinguish between ADD, ADHD, and sensory processing deficits because there is a lot of overlap. One difference; however, explains why children may exhibit a particular behavior. For example, why do some children feel the need to touch everything they see? The difference is that children with ADD or ADHD will do it for the novelty of it. (Example - They will touch everything because it is new to them.) whereas children with an immature sensory system or SPD will do it for the sensation it gives them. (Example - to feel different textures, soft, hard, hot, cold, etc.) So, they are both doing the same thing but to gain different neurological organization or satisfaction from it.

Research has shown that by stimulating the sensory system, primarily through tactile, proprioceptive, and vestibular input, you can make a significant decrease in the sensory seeking or sensory avoiding behaviors seen in kids with ADD and ADHD. A study published in *Science Daily* in 2005 reported that as many as 95% of the children with ADD and ADHD improved with Occupational Therapy treatment—treatment that focused on stimulating or enhancing their sensory system. It is my opinion that pharmacological treatment of ADD and ADHD can be useful for many people. However, I feel that prior to medication, giving children's sensory system a lot of attention may help give many of them the boost that they need. This can enable them to control their behaviors and increase their ability to focus without the need for medication. While medication can do great things, it does have side effects, many of which can be just as hard to deal with as the actual symptoms of ADD and ADHD.

It is important to know that neurobehavioral problems such as ADD and ADHD exist in context. This means that the brain's environment plays an important role and the brain will adapt according to the stimulation it receives. Therefore, ADD and ADHD and attention problems aren't just rooted in the brain. They are directly related to and affected by one's environment. An environment rich in beneficial sensory stimulation can do wonders for the brain. To the contrary, sedentary activities (such as video games and TV watching) don't give children the kind of sensory stimulation that is useful to building their sensory foundation and can take its toll on their neurobehavioral function. For some children the visual input from video games can actually be overstimulating, and for many children the lack of movement they get during these activities can be downright harmful to their development.

For any of you runners who experience the "runner's high" or those of you who know how good you feel after a workout, think about the fact that those same chemicals (dopamine and norepinephrine) are responsible for the "high" that helps children focus. When children exercise and these chemicals are released, their ability to focus increases. This means that enhancing children's environments with opportunities for them to take in the right types of sensory stimulation (especially tactile, proprioceptive, and vestibular) will build their sensory foundation and can enhance their ability to attend and focus.

Let's talk for a minute about the symptoms used in diagnosing ADD and ADHD. According to the American Psychiatric Association's Diagnostic and Statistical Manual, Fifth edition (DSM-5), for the diagnosis of **ADD** to be given to children, they must display six of the following symptoms of inattention for six months or more:

- Often fails to give close attention to details or makes careless mistakes
- Often has difficulty sustaining attention in tasks of play activities
- Often does not listen when spoken to directly
- Often does not follow through on instructions or fails to finish work
- Often has difficulty organizing tasks and activities

- Often avoids, dislikes, or is reluctant to engage in tasks requiring sustained mental effort
- Often loses things
- Often is distracted
- Often is forgetful in daily activities

For a diagnosis of **ADHD**, children must also display six of the symptoms of hyperactivity and impulsivity for more than six months:
- Often fidgets with hands or feet or squirms in seat
- Often has difficulty remaining seated when required to do so
- Often runs or climbs excessively
- Often has difficulty playing quietly
- Often "on the go"
- Often talks excessively
- Often blurts out answers to questions before they have been completed
- Often has difficulty awaiting turn
- Often interrupts or intrudes on others

I want to point out here that these symptoms used to diagnose ADD and ADHD are some of the same symptoms used to describe children with SPD or symptoms that we see in an immature sensory system. Quite often, we use these same criteria when describing children with tactile, proprioceptive, or vestibular immaturity or modulation deficits as many of the symptoms of hyperactivity are seen in children who seek out or crave vestibular or proprioceptive input.

There could be other explanations for these symptoms as well such as food allergies, learning related visual problems, and normal childhood development. Yes! You read that right—normal childhood development. Arnold Gesell, who founded the Yale Clinic of Child Development, reports that these same behaviors listed as criteria for diagnosing ADD and ADHD can be seen in normal children under the age of seven. The Gesell Institute stated in 2005 that "There is an inner timetable which determines the child's rate of development. Trying to teach activities ahead of that timetable will at best result in only minor, temporary growth." It seems as though we live in a society where more and more is being asked of our children at an earlier age. You have to wonder then, if we are labeling our children with diagnoses when they can't live up to these expectations when actually they are just not developmentally ready to meet the demands being placed on them. Practicing a skill over and over again when children are not developmentally ready is not the key, yet we ask four-year-olds to learn to tie shoes, five-year-olds to sit in class for seven hours a day and focus, and six-year-olds to perform on the ball field. We know that skills and habits are not *acquired*, so perhaps the key is building the foundation which will allow children to *develop* the skills needed to tie shoes, sit and focus in the classroom, or to be able to perform on the ball field.

> "Everybody is a GENIUS. But if you judge a fish by its ability to climb a tree, it will live its whole life believing that it is stupid." ~ Albert Einstein

There is a quote by Albert Einstein that I love because I feel it speaks right to that point. He states, "Everybody is a genius. But if you judge a fish by its ability to climb a tree, it will live its whole life believing that it is stupid." When we ask our kids to perform skills ahead of their developmental timeline, we put them at risk for losing confidence and giving up.

I want to also touch on visual problems as being something that can look a lot like ADD or ADHD. I have seen this countless times in my experience as an OT. Children may have 20/20 eyesight but good vision is more than just good eyesight. Vision includes oculomotor skills, visual processing, visual perceptual skills, visual motor skills, and even the ability to visualize. Many kids are lacking in one or more of these areas and this can make focusing on academic work quite challenging. I will give you an example of a fifth grade boy named Cole who came to me but also had a psychoeducational testing scheduled for the following week to help determine if he had ADHD (which his parents and teachers were suspecting). Upon oculomotor testing, I realized that he sees double. For him, this was all he knew so he didn't realize there was anything different. Can you imagine? Fifth grade and this boy had been seeing double his whole life and trying to focus on his academics only to seem to fail at doing so. I referred Cole to a developmental optometrist who could do a typical eye exam but then do further testing as needed to dig deeper. What Cole needed was vision therapy. Voila! Cole's ADHD symptoms disappeared.

I can give you countless examples just like Cole's but what I want to stress here is that if your child has signs such as difficulty focusing, difficulty with or a dislike of reading, difficulty with ball skills, difficulty with handwriting, or other signs that could be associated with vision, take them to a developmental optometrist in your area to check that off your list prior to having them tested for ADD or ADHD.

Neil's Story

I want to tell you about an eight-year-old boy named Neil whom I worked with. Neil came to me for handwriting help, but I quickly discovered that poor handwriting was just a symptom of other deficits he had that fell under the sensory processing umbrella. Neil had been diagnosed with ADHD at some point earlier in his life and was taking medication for this at the time I was working with him. What I noticed right away with Neil were a couple of obvious signs that his sensory cup was not full and he was trying so hard to get it there. He unfortunately often chose to do this in inappropriate ways.

I noticed Neil chewing on my business card as he sat in the waiting room. I later discovered that he would chew a sucker as soon as he put it in his mouth (never licking it) and that he was a "shirt chewer" with a constant wet ring around his collar. He had poor trunk strength and had to brace himself with one hand on the wall while using his other hand to write on the chalkboard. He also demonstrated poor trunk control and strength as he used his tongue during any activity that required trunk control. It is not uncommon for children with decreased trunk strength and postural control/stability to stick their tongues out when their core strength is being challenged. The reason for this being that oral-motor control comes from good trunk and neck control. If those two things are not present, you may start to see the child compensate for poor trunk control with the oral-motor activity of sticking their tongue out. They may do this while jumping on the trampoline or working to maintain good upright posture while seated at their desk to write.

I noticed something else with Neil that told me that his trunk control and postural stability were lacking. I noticed that it was nearly impossible for him to sit up in a desk while doing his work. He would slump over his work putting his head within inches of his paper. This was a quick indicator to me that not only was there a problem with his vestibular and proprioceptive foundation but that he may also struggle with the reflex portion of his building blocks of learning and that some of his infant reflexes may not have fully matured. After further observation and discussions with his mother, I soon realized that while Neil may have ADHD, he was also struggling with a great deal of sensory under responsiveness. Neil was not functioning at his optimum level of arousal, and he was seeking out movement to try to fill his sensory cup in order to get him there. Whether or not ADHD was truly an accurate diagnosis for him, one thing was very clear to me, he needed a lot of work on his sensory system and reflex integration and did not have a broad enough foundation of his building blocks of learning. This was starting to have terrible effects on him as the demands placed on him in school got greater and greater.

Josh's Story

Now let me tell you about another eight-year-old boy, this one whose name is Josh. Josh's second grade teacher told his parents that she suspects Josh has ADD. She noticed that Josh had a hard time staying focused, following through on instructions, finishing his work, and had difficulty when it came to self-organization and organization of his school work. Josh's parents were surprised to hear this but knew their son was struggling so were happy to know that they had possibly found the answer. The problem was, however, that they truly did not feel that their son had ADD so they were reluctant to talk to his doctor about this.

Josh's mom is a friend of mine so we started discussing everything that was going on with him and the behaviors that were putting up the red flags. What I found out was that Josh was eight and walked on his tiptoes. Josh had poor balance and was unable to ride a bike without training wheels. He was incredibly sensitive to loud noises. She told me that Josh complained of being tired a lot and had poor endurance, which was especially noticeable on the soccer field. Josh also still sucked his thumb and chewed his shirts until they had a wet ring around the collar, and sometimes even chewed holes in them. Josh had recently started using scissors to cut his shirt while seated at his desk and had been cutting up other objects in his desk during class time. She told me that Josh was not a coordinated child, had difficulty learning new motor skills, and his handwriting was just one of the things that suffered because of that. Josh was far from hyperactive and was often described as "laid back" because he preferred sedentary activities.

After talking to his mom and gathering this information, it became clear to me that while Josh had symptoms consistent with ADD, he also had a great deal of symptoms consistent with an immature sensory system and that had sensory modulation deficits. What stood out to me the most was the fact that he was quite possibly seeking out proprioceptive input through sucking his thumb and walking on his tiptoes. Hearing that he had poor balance, poor coordination, fatigued easily, and preferred sedentary activities also signaled to me that he had vestibular deficits. My advice to her was to start with Occupational Therapy and taking a closer look at his sensory system prior to pursuing the medication route.

Paul's Story

Let me share another story about a nine-year-old boy named Paul. Paul struggles to stay tuned-in in class. He always seems to be one step behind the others. His grades are good, but his behaviors are impulsive, he lacks organizational skills, and he is easily distracted. These behaviors seem to cause

Paul to get in to trouble quite often. His teachers have told his parents that they think he has ADHD. Not knowing what else to do, Paul's parents talked to his pediatrician. His parents went down the diagnostic criteria checklist for ADHD, and sure enough, he met the criteria for diagnosis and was started on medication. Paul's mom came to me and explained that she and Paul's dad just really didn't feel this was the answer and that ADHD wasn't truly what was causing him these difficulties. After talking with her and learning more about Paul, I realized he has sensory under responsiveness in his tactile, proprioceptive, and vestibular senses. Paul was just never functioning at an optimum level of arousal. Every day was like a Monday morning to him. How could he focus and control his behaviors? He was not at an optimum level. His cup was never getting filled.

Within weeks of working with Paul and his parents and giving them strategies to help him fill his cup and reach his optimum level of arousal, they noticed a difference. He was more interactive with them, was less likely to fly off the handle over a situation with his sister, could handle being in unfamiliar situations better, and was overall doing so much better, and without his ADHD medication. They worked hard each day to fill his cup and keep it filled. They used an exercise ball for lying on, rocking on, and punching. He started off his day kicking a soccer ball against a wall or jumping on a trampoline. He would crab walk or wheelbarrow around the house. His mom would pull him around the floor of the house on a blanket and spin him. When she saw things getting hairy, she would have him stop and do push-ups and jumping jacks. She was amazed that in the few seconds it took for him to do jumping jacks and push-ups, he was totally transformed. He could sit and focus again after doing so. His mom told me that she would have him use some of his sensory strategies prior to activities such as piano lessons. She said that typically he would have to go in and touch everything prior to starting and that he was very fidgety. With a few sensory strategies, his cup got filled prior to his lesson starting, and he no longer acted in that way. Paul became more open and social with me and appeared more confident. Best of all, his parents were relieved that they knew what to do for him and they could see how much better he was doing.

Neil, Josh, and Paul, like so many other kids, have symptoms that fall under the ADD/ADHD diagnostic criteria but also are consistent with an immature sensory system and in some cases sensory processing disorder, and specifically Sensory Modulation Disorder. They can't sit still, are distracted, can't focus, and are disorganized because their sensory cups aren't filled to the right level in order to provide the opportunity for them to be at their optimum level of arousal. They are seeking out movement and, until they get enough and get their cup filled, they will continue to seek out movement. They will move, fidget, wiggle, bounce off the walls, stare into outer space, be one step behind the rest of the class, seem as if they aren't with it, and simply have a hard time focusing.

Proper diagnosis is vital for the treatment of ADD and ADHD because, while medication can be wonderful for some children, medicating for the wrong thing can be detrimental. It is my opinion that we should START WITH THE SENSORY FOUNDATION before we medicate since we know that treatment focused on stimulating or enhancing children's sensory systems can greatly improve the symptoms of ADD and ADHD. Again, this is my opinion and you know your children better than anybody. As my pediatrician always told me, "Go with your gut." If you and your children's doctor feel medication is needed, do it. BUT, work on their sensory foundation in conjunction with the medication. Build their sensory foundation so that medication may not have to be the long term solution. If your gut tells you that ADD or ADHD may not be the only thing going on here, do your own "investigation." Work to figure out whether perhaps your children just aren't functioning at their optimum level of arousal because their sensory system is immature, if they have sensory integration dysfunction, or if their sensory cup isn't where it needs to be.

Recognizing that children with ADD or ADHD demonstrate sensory processing deficits is key to helping us know how to help them. We need to provide:

- Interventions to help them build their sensory foundation (specifically their proprioceptive, vestibular, and tactile foundations). (Refer to chapters 23, 24, and 25.)
- Strategies to help them to self-regulate and gain self-awareness. (Refer to chapter 29 for self-regulation/calming strategies.)
- Sensory strategies to help them achieve their optimum level of arousal, thereby increasing their ability to focus and engage in a task. Use the sensory check-list in appendix A to help you determine your children's over and under sensitivities. Then refer to chapters 26 and 27 for strategies to use to fill their cups or remedy an overflowing cup to help them reach their optimum level of arousal.

CHAPTER 17

AUTISM SPECTRUM DISORDER AND THE SENSORY SYSTEM

There are many great resources with wonderful information regarding autism spectrum disorder (ASD). What I want to touch on here is not in-depth information regarding symptoms and diagnoses; instead, I want to give you some insight into how ASD ties in to the sensory system and how sensory strategies can be used to help these children.

First, let's talk about why autism is referred to as the autism spectrum. Autism is referred to as a spectrum disorder because the symptoms, skills, level of impairment, or disability can vary greatly from a mild impairment to a severe impairment. All children on the autism spectrum will have some of these core symptoms in the following three areas:

- **Social impairment**
  - Difficulty forming and maintaining relationships with their peers
  - Difficulty sharing emotions and understanding how others think and feel. They may have trouble identifying their own emotions.
  - Difficulty holding a conversation
  - Difficulty interacting with the people around them, thus often playing by themselves vs. interacting with the group of kids
  - Often described as socially "awkward"

- **Spoken and Unspoken Communication**
  - Slow to develop language and perhaps did not babble as an infant
  - Use of one word answers
  - Tendency to repeat the same phrases over and over
  - Avoid making eye contact
  - Slow to develop the use of gestures such as pointing, showing things to others, and smiling (perhaps fail altogether to do this)

- Difficulty starting and maintaining a conversation and learning to take turns in a conversation
- Have difficulty understanding a joke or may take sarcastic comments literally
- May have flat speech that lacks tone, pitch, and accent

- **Repetitive/stereotyped behaviors** (may be extreme and noticeable or mild and discreet)
    - Inflexibility with the need to follow a strict schedule or routine
    - Repetitive motions such as flapping their arms, walking in specific patterns, hair twirling
    - Have very specific areas of interests (often in numbers, symbols, or science)
    - May become fascinated with parts of objects (for example, the wheels of their cars) and spend hours lining up their cars or trains vs. playing with them
    - Have an overwhelming preoccupation with a subject matter such as animals or cars and will choose only to talk about and play with items that fall under that preoccupation
    - May not do well with changes to their environment (such as changing the décor or a paint color, mom wearing her hair different, sleeping in a different bed on vacation, etc.)

Symptoms of autism are present at birth; however, they can be difficult to notice during infancy. It is usually during the toddler years that parents and caregivers start to notice symptoms as they have problems with language development and their lack of interaction (and desire for interaction) with others. While most children with autism may be slow in gaining new knowledge or skills, and may have a lower than normal level of intelligence, there are children with autism who have normal to high intelligence (even though they may have trouble communicating or applying what they know).

While the number of children being diagnosed with autism spectrum disorder (ASD) is increasing, the good news is that the numbers of these children showing us that they can overcome, compensate for, and manage the challenges of autism is also increasing. It is important to understand the connection that these diagnoses have with the sensory system since sensory integration may just be the most difficult aspect of ASD to understand but may also be the most crucial. Chantal

Sicile-Kira, the author of the book Autism Life Skills (2008), writes that in her research of adults who fall anywhere on the autism spectrum, sensory processing challenges were the number one struggle they faced as children and that impacted their relationships, communication, self-awareness, safety and so on. "Tribe (1992)...claimed that 'there is enough evidence to suggest that sensory processing impairment is as central to autism as the impairments of social interaction, communication, and imagination" (Talay-Ongan & Wood, 2000).

In the book Movement and Action in Learning and Development (Stockman, 2004), the author writes that children's experiences and interactions with the world should be given the same consideration as limits in their biological makeup. Many children with ASD, for example, have a disconnect between the brain and their tactile, vestibular, and proprioceptive senses, the senses that involve movement and our physical interaction with the world. Movement is connected to the way we perceive and interpret the world around us and plays a role in how we learn. For these kids "normal" learning seems to be limited by this disconnect as well as their lack of collaboration between all of their other senses.

For children on the autism spectrum, the way they perceive the world around them through their senses is distorted. This means that what may seem like an ordinary smell, sight, sound, touch, movement, or taste to you and me may go unnoticed or seem threatening or painful to them. Let's consider for a moment all of the sensations that children experience simply being in their own home (the one place that should be our place of refuge).

- Think about the **visual overstimulation** children may get from the bright lights from lamps or overhead lights, bright sunlight streaming in through the windows, the constantly changing picture on the TV, bright light from computer screens, home decor, brightly colored furniture or accessories, toys lying around, moving ceiling fans, moving bodies, or clutter on the counters.
- Think about the **auditory overstimulation** children may get from dogs barking, the doorbell ringing, the sounds coming from the radio or the TV (not to mention, both turned on at the same time), kids yelling, mom and dad talking (and sometimes loudly), several conversations going on at one time, the air conditioner running, the washer and dryer, the fan on the stove blowing, the phone ringing, or water running.
- Think about the **overstimulation from smells** such as air fresheners, laundry detergent, flowers, mom's perfume, dad's cologne, dinner

cooking, coffee brewing, odors from pets, scented candles, scented soaps, or those that come from cleaning products.

This is just the tip of the iceberg. Think about the sights, smells, sounds, and movements that can overstimulate children on what seems like a simple car ride, trip to the grocery store, or dinner out at a restaurant. Can you understand why children with autism may frequently have meltdowns or tantrums? Their senses have been overloaded, and they are trying to communicate that to you the best way they know how. Knowing this is the first step. When you realize what is going on you can work to eliminate some of these stimuli or know ahead of time what kind of situation may arise and use some preventative measures. Shore (2004) stated that "understanding the paradigm that people perceive the world differently is vital for working successfully with people on the autism spectrum."

It has been stated that as many as 90% of individuals with autism spectrum disorder (ASD) have sensory processing dysfunction. (Baranek et al., 2006; Leekamet al., 2007; Tomchek and Dunn, 2007; Baker et al., 2008). These children have difficulty regulating their responses to sensory stimuli which can lead to behaviors and responses that can be hard to predict. Not only that but they can often vary dramatically from one situation to another. In Chapter 10, I explained that how we register sensory input and how our level of arousal is affected are deeply connected. It makes sense then that children with ASD will have trouble reaching and maintaining an optimum level of arousal. Children with ASD are also at risk for anxiety and depression as they struggle to deal with and sort out the sensory input that is all around them.

I mentioned earlier the three domains in which children with ASD struggle: communication, socialization, and repetitive or stereotyped behaviors. Evidence suggests that impairments in these areas can be linked to poor sensory processing. For example, the stereotyped and repetitive behaviors these children sometimes exhibit may serve to neurologically organize them. Behaviors such as flapping their arms or walking in the same repetitive path may provide the sensory input they need to satisfy their sensory under or over-responsiveness or sensitivity. Stephen Shore (2003), an adult with ASD, describes his difficulty in socialization due to his sensory over-responsiveness. He writes that as a toddler he could not tolerate kissing his dad because of the scratchiness of his moustache and the smell of coffee on his breath. He also states that he could never work at a job where wearing a suit was required. He found suits and ties to be so uncomfortable that wearing one would keep him from being able to perform his job.

What researchers are trying to uncover is what comes first - the chicken or the egg? Do children with ASD have sensory processing problems because of their limited interaction with their environment? Or, perhaps, is it that they do not engage in their environment because of their poor sensory processing skills? Either way, we know that interaction with the environment and the sensory stimulation that this provides them is important and these children may not be getting enough of it.

While this cause and effect relationship between sensory processing and environment is yet unproven, what is documented is children's improvement in the areas of communication, socialization, and repetitive/stereotyped behaviors as a response to sensory processing intervention . . . and I see it every day. Not only do I see it, but parents see it too. When we pay close attention to children's sensory systems and their over and under responsivities and then work to give them what their sensory systems need, great results follow. This work can help children with ASD to process sensory input and then learn to respond appropriately.

I want to include a statement from an article written by Jim Chapman (a father who has two sons with ASD). He writes about the effectiveness of therapies (and specifically sensory integration therapy) on children with ASD. Chapman writes, "When my wife came home and told me that the occupational therapist (OTR) wanted us to perform 'joint compressions and brushing every two hours' on our youngest son, my response was essentially, 'That's the craziest thing I have ever heard.' After overcoming my initial objections, I quickly became a believer when I observed the dramatic changes in our son's behavior and in his ability to adapt to various situations."

Recognizing that children with ASD demonstrate sensory processing deficits (and specifically sensory modulation deficits) is key to helping us understand what types of intervention to provide for these children. We know that we need to provide:

- Interventions to help them build their sensory foundation (specifically their proprioceptive, vestibular, and tactile foundations) so they can learn to respond appropriately to the sensory information they receive from the world around them. (Refer to chapters 23, 24, and 25.)
- Strategies to help them with transitions from one setting to another, one person to another, and to help them to self-regulate. Children with ASD are often very visual so we focus on visual strategies such as picture schedules and picture books with calming strategies from

which they may choose. Using deep pressure activities and other tactile, proprioceptive, and vestibular strategies that are calming can be very helpful. (Refer to chapter 29 for self-regulation/calming strategies).

- Sensory strategies to help increase their level of arousal, thereby increasing their ability to focus and engage in a task or social encounter. Use the sensory check-list (appendix A) to help you determine your children's over and under sensitivities. Then refer to chapters 26 and 27 for strategies to use to fill their cups or remedy an "overflowing cup" to help them reach their optimum level of arousal.

CHAPTER 18

FEARS, ANXIETY, MELTDOWNS, OR DIFFICULTY WITH TRANSITIONS

The emotional behaviors that we see in our children can oftentimes alarm us or worry us the most and are often what lead parents to seek out help in the first place. That is why I want to take some time explaining why we see some of these emotional behaviors in our children. Again, when you understand why, you can get to the root of the problem and work on fixing it versus just putting a Band-Aid on it (or even worse, thinking you just have a bad kid).

When children have trouble processing the sensory information that they receive from the world around them, it is very common for them to have fears and anxiety. Let's go back to the building blocks of learning again and remember that emotional and behavioral regulation is at the top of the building blocks and is an area of performance in which we can see children struggle. All kids are going to have their moments where they throw temper tantrums, hit, cry, scream, and are inconsolable. Heck, we all do. We all can get a little crazy when we are feeling bombarded or overwhelmed. When children have difficulty taking in,

> When children have trouble processing the sensory information that they receive from the world around them, it is very common for them to have FEARS and ANXIETY.

making sense out of, and adapting to the sensory information they receive every moment of every day, you may see them reach this state more often and at times when you wouldn't expect it. They may have difficulty coping and show signs of anger, aggression, withdrawal, anxiety, depression, or hostility. Poor emotional regulation can also lead to difficulty with focusing and attending and may make children appear hyperactive or distractible.

Why does this happen? Well, there can be several different explanations:

- **An overflowing sensory cup** – I have explained the problems that children who are over- sensitive to sensory input or whose sensory cups are overflowing may face. Children who are overly sensitive to sensory stimuli, who experience a situation in which their sensory systems get flooded or their sensory cups start overflowing may kick in to "fight, flight, or fright" mode. Remember that what is happening is that their sensory system perceives something that to you or me may seem like a normal, unthreatening stimulus, but their sensory system perceives it as noxious or threatening. The stimulus that makes them react this way may not be one that we would ever think would have this effect on them but may lead them to act out emotionally, aggressively, or become quite anxious.

    I often ask parents to look at what is taking place around the children at the time of a meltdown or to look at what has taken place just prior. Often, you will discover that your children might have been in a situation where their sensory cup was filled to the brim and now something caused it to overflow. Perhaps, they play well with another child one on one but do not play well with others in a group setting. If we read into that, it may be the overstimulation from the group that causes the meltdown, tantrum, etc. Perhaps there are very bright lights, loud sounds, strong smells, lots of commotion, etc. that cause your children's cup to overflow. One example that I see often is a fear of the bathroom at the clinic. I have kids meltdown and downright refuse to go in. Why??? The hand dryer is incredibly loud and the flushing of the toilet. Two loud and *unpredictable* sounds. A huge trigger for many kids is a long day at school or other crowded situations with lots of people and sounds. When you know this, you can help by preparing them ahead of time with calming strategies or working to eliminate any of the overwhelming sensory input that is within your control.

- **Changes in routine or environment** – When children's sensory systems are immature or if they have difficulty modulating the sensory information they receive, they will often need a routine with no unexpected changes to it. If they are used to going straight home after school, having a snack, and having playtime and you change this up, you may rock their world. Let's say you decide to run an errand on the way home from school and have them eat a snack in the car. This seems like a pretty reasonable request, right? Well, not to some kids. Other changes that may rock their world could be a substitute teacher, changing the color of their room or home décor, changing what you pack in their lunchbox, etc. When children have predictability, they feel in control and feel comfortable and safe with what is going on around them. They know they will not need to adapt to any new sensory input, and they will do anything to keep things constant. If their day is predictable, they can prepare their sensory system for what it is going to have to deal with. If you change that, they don't know what to expect or what new sensory input they may receive that could be hard for them to handle and they may become anxious, fearful, or emotional because of this. This can be why transitioning from one activity to another is challenging for some. They may not be ready to adapt to the new activity or situation and the sensory challenges that it entails.

- **Being stuck in an immature emotional pattern** – According to Doreit Bailer and Lucy Jane Miller (2011), children will get stuck in an immature pattern of handling emotions rather than maturing in the way that they do so. Think about the differences in how we cope as we grow and mature from infancy to adulthood. Children with sensory processing problems may use the same strategies in a difficult situation that you see in much younger children such as hitting, crying, biting, relying on a caregiver for comfort, etc. instead of being able to identify the emotion, talk about it, and negotiate a solution to their problem.

- **Experiencing the unexpected** – As I mentioned above in changes in routine or environment, fears and anxieties are often present because children are afraid of what unexpected sensory input they are going to have to deal with. Let's use the school bus for example. I can't tell you how many kids with whom I have worked have a lot of trouble associated with the school bus and often just refuse to get on it. Think about it. The school bus is one of the most sensory overloading activities children will ever face. Unexpected bumps, starts, stops, kids brushing up against them as they walk to their seats, screaming kids, sirens, and so on. Not to mention, they are riding the bus at the beginning of the day when they may still be groggy and haven't gotten their sensory cup to its optimum level yet or at the end of the day when their cup is on the brink of overflowing, and they are tired from a long day. The cafeteria with its smells, noises, kids touching them, etc. can also have the same effect on children as the school bus. This setting has so much sensory stimulation and so much of it is unexpected and out of children's control. Situations like these can quite frequently cause fear and anxiety.

In the same way, a big party, a trip to your local big-box store, an outing to a movie theater, a new restaurant, etc. can cause fear and anxiety as well. The smell of popcorn, food, or lumber, the sounds coming from crying babies, loud hand dryers, or people talking unexpectedly over a loudspeaker, unfamiliar people wanting to strike up a conversation, being asked to play with toys with which they have never played, or partaking in an unfamiliar activity can be quite overwhelming. It is nearly impossible for children to feel in control in these situations and that can be scary, especially to someone whose sensory cup is at its threshold, is about to bubble over or someone who is functioning in a state of overarousal.

The point I am trying to drive home here is for you to think about *what* is going on in your children's environment that may make them act the way they are acting. Consider *which* of their senses may be being overloaded and *why* this particular situation makes them act the way they do? It will be a lot easier to help your children if you can get to the root of the problem. Do they need more or less of a certain sensory input? Which of the children's sensory cups are overflowing, and how can I work to balance that out? Knowing the answers to these questions will help you problem solve and figure out how you can help. Look at their sensory foundation as a possible cause and let part of the solution be to build their sensory foundation. Refer to the activities listed in chapters 23, 24, and 25 for help to do just that. In the meantime, what every parent, teacher, or caregiver needs is a bag of tricks to use during those very moments. There are many strategies we can use to help them cope and learn to self-regulate their emotions. (Refer to chapter 29 for a list of and explanation of these strategies.)

CHAPTER 19

GROWTH SPURTS = REGRESSION

I'm now going to take a departure from quoting research and talking about diagnoses. I am going to throw in my own opinion or theory based on what I see through my experiences working with kids, what I hear about when talking to other parents, and what I live day-to-day as a mother. I think you will able to follow me and probably relate to what I am going to say.

Do you ever find that as your children make great leaps in development in one area, they may regress in another? Or perhaps when they hit a growth spurt, do you find they take a few steps back in other areas? For example, maybe they all of a sudden develop the gross motor skill to make it all the way across the monkey bars without your help, the fine motor skills to tie their shoes, showing never before seen skills and creativity when drawing, start sounding words out as they develop their pre-reading skills, and start being able to add and subtract and doing some simple math. Wow! That is a lot of physical and cognitive development for children to handle. Or maybe they start a new school year and you see them all of a sudden start bursting with new knowledge. But, uh oh! What happened to my children who didn't talk back, didn't get in to much trouble, and seemed to obey the rules? In case you can't tell, I'm writing from experience. This is what our family experienced when my son was 5 ½ years old. It wasn't the first time, either. Throughout my son's life, I've noticed that he may make great strides developmentally but then seems to regress in other areas. He becomes fearful of things he wasn't fearful of, he starts testing limits he never tested before, has tantrums for no reason, or just can't seem to pull himself together sometimes. It's not just my son either. My daughter who had never sucked her thumb or took a pacifier as an infant started chewing on her shirt, her hand, her arm, and whatever else she can get her hands on and "W-sitting." How can this be?

I want you to picture the building blocks of learning again, remembering that it is strategically shaped like a pyramid. It is shaped like a pyramid because the layers at the bottom need to be broader than the blocks at the top to give it stability and a firm foundation. What I believe happens as children develop, and especially when they make these sudden leaps in development, is that their foundation suffers. The building blocks get so top-heavy from a gain in development in the performance areas that the foundation just isn't adequate anymore. As their motor skills and performance take off and get bigger in size (the top of the building), the foundation of the building blocks loses some ground. When this happens, I believe children then need a revamping of their foundation. Their building blocks look more like a rectangle and need to be reshaped to regain its triangular shape. The foundation needs to be strengthened to be made sturdy again.

This change would explain why my son all of a sudden had to climb on everything that was standing still or jump on the trampoline every chance he got (and often the furniture when he didn't think I am looking). He was seeking out proprioception to build that part of his foundation. He couldn't get enough of swinging on the playset in our backyard. He longed for the vestibular input that gives. That behavior also explained why he asked to chew gum from the time he woke up in the morning until the time he went to bed. Luckily his teeth didn't rot out. He was craving the proprioceptive input that those heavy work muscles of his mouth got when chewing. This would also explain why my daughter started chewing on things as she was also craving proprioceptive input. I don't want to forget to mention, also, that my son started sleeping with his soft blanket that he used as a baby but hadn't asked to use for 2 ½ years. He wanted that soft tactile input.

Along with sensory seeking behaviors, what I also saw was that he was emotionally regressing as his building blocks were taking on a new look and adjustments were being made to the blocks. Remember that at the top of the building blocks is a block for emotional and behavioral regulation. What I noticed was that he was much more sensitive, all of a sudden, and would cry or become so emotionally distraught over the slightest thing. He would let the smallest disagreement with his sister or an episode of not getting what he wanted totally lead him to a meltdown. You could almost see it in his eyes. He was so disorganized mentally that he didn't really know what to do with himself; consequently, his emotional self-regulation suffered.

My son is lucky enough (or unlucky enough) to have an Occupational Therapist for a mom and one who analyzes everything he does. As I analyzed his behaviors, I realized that because his foundation had weakened and his sensory system had taken a hit as a result of the effort going into the top of his building blocks, he was seeking out input to his sensory system. This quite possibly was his own subconscious attempt to strengthen his foundation. That is when I had to kick n to full OT mom mode. I realized that I could either try to reason with him all day long and get absolutely nowhere, or I could use the strategies I knew would neurologically organize him. When he would get into that irrational meltdown mode, I quickly started spinning him in a swivel chair (vestibular input), picked up his feet to make him walk on his hands to do the "wheelbarrow" (proprioceptive input), and gave him a deep bear hug (more proprioceptive input). Or I would take him aside and let him lie on his tummy while I rolled a rubber kickball up and down his back firmly, or I would quickly offer him bubble gum or a drink with a straw for sucking (again, more deep pressure/proprioceptive input). See chapters 23, 24, and 25 for a more comprehensive list of strategies you can utilize.

The thing that I have always had to remind myself throughout the years is that it is just a phase and as soon as his pyramid takes shape again and after he learns to adjust to all of the developmental changes he is going through, I will get my son back!

SECTION 3 - THERE IS HOPE:

HOW TO HELP YOUR CHILDREN

CHAPTER 20

THE BRAIN CAN CHANGE

I want to explain neuroplasticity briefly because without it there would be no help for our children. Without neuroplasticity, I would not have a job, and this book would not exist. This is because neuroplasticity is what allows our brains to change. It is neuroplasticity that gives us hope that we can help our children develop and grow and make a difference in their lives. What a beautiful thing that we were created with the ability for our brains to grow and change when given the tools to do so. If our children's foundations couldn't be changed, if no amount of exercise or all of the strategies in the world could change their performance and behaviors, then it would be time to give up hope. It is because of neuroplasticity; however, that we have the ability to grow our children's foundations and increase their chances of success. I am about to get technical here, so bare with me for just a minute.

> It is NEUROPLASTICITY that gives us hope that we can help our children develop and grow and make a difference in their lives.

The human brain has neuroplasticity, meaning it can reorganize itself by forming new neural connections throughout life based on experiences. Neuroplasticity is the ability of the brain to change with learning - the kind of learning that occurs through instruction or experience.

The brain is shaped by the characteristics of a person's *environment* and by that person's *actions*. Following birth, newborns' brains are flooded with information from their sense organs. This information has to make it to the brain where it can be processed. This requires nerve cells (or neurons) to make connections with one another to transmit the impulses to the brain. The newborn's genes instruct the pathway to the correct area of the brain from a particular nerve cell. For example, nerve cells in the eye send impulses to the visual area of the brain and not to the area of the brain that is responsible for speech and language. This process continues over the first few years of life and infants' and toddlers' brains grow quickly. Maturation continues and an increasing number of synaptic connections are made. According to Gopnick, et al, (1999), at birth, each nerve cell in the brain has approximately 2,500 synapses and by the time the infant reaches its toddler years, the number of synapses is approximately 15,000 per nerve cell.

The number of synapses decreases as we age through a process called synaptic pruning. Synaptic pruning is the process of eliminating weaker synaptic connections while the stronger connections are kept and strengthened. Experiences are what will determine which connections will be pruned and which ones will be strengthened. The connections used the most are the ones that are preserved. Neurons must have a purpose to survive. Without purpose neurons will die.

Plasticity enables the process of developing and pruning connections which, in turn, allows the brain to adapt to the environment. To put this in to simpler terms, our neural connections will be strengthened when they are used and challenged. I think about how bad I am at math now compared to how good I was at it when I was a child. Math was my strongest subject, and I actually tested in to a pretty high-level math class in college (I'm not bragging though). Now, not so much. My dog may be better at math than me now. Why did I go from mathematician to barely being able to add 2+2? It is because I don't use math anymore. I imagine that if I had a scan done of my brain, it would show that a lot of my math synapses have been pruned. The good news is that while I am no mathematician anymore, I have become better at other things and strengthened other areas of my brain (At least I'd like to think). Have you ever heard the saying, "If you don't use it you'll lose it."? That is very true when it comes to neuroplasticity and we have to help kids find ways to "use it."

Neuroplasticity has such profound implications for all children whether they are "typically" developing, have an immature sensory system, or have a diagnosis. All children can improve the ability of their brain to efficiently receive and process information. According to *www.learningbreakthrough.com*, any time children learn to do something new, are confronted by a stimulus they haven't experienced before, or adapt to the demands of their environment, their brains develop further. The website also states that activities that promote balance and spatial awareness specifically (think vestibular and proprioceptive input) have a profound effect on higher brain functions like reading, math, memory, and comprehension. What is also interesting is that studies show that increasing the level of difficulty of an activity increases the number of neurons or nerve cells that the brain must use to fulfill the demands of the activity.

Now that you, hopefully, have a clearer picture of neuroplasticity and what it means, you realize how important it is to provide our children with the sensory stimulation that is vital to building their sensory foundation. Receiving this sensory stimulation will increase their ability to take in, organize, and act according to the sensations received from the world around them. When we provide our children with challenges, we can greatly increase the brain's efficiency by increasing its neural involvement. How exciting! We get to become "plastic" surgeons as we help our children's brains grow and develop.

So, in a nutshell, neuroplasticity is a fancy word but can be summarized like this: Our brain has the ability to change and grow. To quote Marvin L. Minsky (*Society of the Mind,* 1986), "The principle activities of brains are making changes in themselves." Good thing! It would be disheartening to think I could never better myself from where I am at right now.

CHAPTER 21

A FEW SENSORY QUESTIONS TO ASK YOURSELF

I know you are getting sick of me saying this, but I want to stress again how important it is that when you see problems in your child's performance or emotional control, you begin looking at the sensory foundation and the sensory system to get to the root of the problem. Now, as you are trying to put everything together based on the information I have given, I want to give you a few questions that you can ask yourself to help you do just that, get to the root of the problem:

- Does my child seem to avoid certain items or situations; if so, what sensory stimuli are involved that is making my child want to avoid it? For example, does my child try to avoid going to the movie theater? Could this be because of the loud noises?
- Are certain situations sure to cause my child to have a meltdown and could the meltdown be caused by sensory stimulation involved with that situation? For example, does my child seem to always have a meltdown after a birthday party, in a crowded situation, or before or after getting on the school bus?
- Does my child seem to seek out or crave certain things or movements; if so, what sensory system is involved? For example, does my child constantly need to be climbing, touching things, or moving? If so, your child is showing you that he or she needs extra proprioceptive, tactile, or vestibular input.
- Could my child be in "fight, flight, or fright" mode? Is my child biting, hitting, running, or having a tantrum in response to certain situations or sensory stimuli? For example, does he or she become aggressive in response to touch or certain textures (including food textures)?
- Do many of my child's fears or anxieties seem to relate to an event or activity that may pertain to a sensory system? For example, is there a fear of haircuts, messy hands, swinging, or not having both feet on the ground?

A FEW SENSORY QUESTIONS TO ASK YOURSELF

- Does my child seem to avoid or meltdown in situations that involve a change in routine or that would create a situation where he or she cannot control the sensory input received? For example, does a substitute teacher throw my child way off? Is vacation and adjusting to new surroundings difficult? Does my child have a hard time adjusting when there is a change in the order of the daily routine?
- Is it possible that my child cannot sit still and focus because movement is needed to help get neurologically organized in order to focus?
- Does my child seem to lack organizational skills or the ability to fully participate in school, with peers, or in extracurricular activities due to not being at that optimum level arousal? Does my child seem to be functioning in an under aroused (Monday morning-like) state?
- What is it that my child consistently seeks out or avoids?

When you learn to ask yourself these questions and have the tools to answer them, you will be better equipped to properly address what is going on. If your child has a severe dislike of certain food textures and also hates having messy hands, you can start to realize that your child may have an oversensitivity to tactile stimulation and could use a boost in that area. If your child cannot sit still to focus on learning tasks and seems to love to jump, fidget, and play hard, you can put the pieces of the puzzle together that your child is craving extra proprioceptive and vestibular input. You can then work to provide activities that will supply that throughout your child's day and especially prior to those times when sitting still is going to be required. When your child is having a meltdown, think of what calming activities you can provide. If you know that your child is going to become overstimulated by a birthday party or time at the play area of your local fast food restaurants, you can automatically put some calming activities in to place as soon as you get home and even in the car.

As I mentioned earlier, when you know why you are seeing certain behaviors in your child or why he or she is struggling in certain areas, you can equip yourself and your child with the tools needed to help. Refer to chapters 23-29 to help you put together a bag of tricks to help you do just that. This will help you to enhance your child's sensory system in order to achieve greater self-regulation and emotional or behavioral control. This will also help with skill development for greater success in curricular or extracurricular activities which can aid in improving self-esteem. These strategies can be used to help ANY child.

CHAPTER 22

WORKING SENSORY INPUT IN TO AN ALREADY BUSY DAY

Hopefully, by now you understand how important it is to provide frequent opportunities for your children to receive sensory input. If you are like I would be, you may be wondering "How in the world am I going to work this into our already very busy day?" The bad news is that every 30 minutes children should receive some sort of tactile, proprioceptive, or vestibular input. Don't let that stress you though. The good news is that it is easy to accomplish this, and you don't have to spend a lot of time or money. The key is to make it a part of your family's lifestyle. Build opportunities for your children to get sensory input into their everyday activities. Trust me. I get it, I am a busy parent, too, and the last thing I want is something added to my already very full plate. You have my guarantee that these things can be done with just minimal extra effort and they do work. These techniques have all been mom tested and kid-approved.

Let me warn you, though, we have to be OK with our houses (or maybe just a room or two) looking a little more like playland and a little less orderly. We need to encourage movement and discourage sedentary activities. We need to let our kids get messy and explore the world around them. We have to use our judgment, of course, but put aside some of our irrational fears and let our kids move and be kids. I worked with a little boy who was 5-years-old and preparing for kindergarten. His parents were concerned because he couldn't bear to be away from mom and had never been left with a babysitter or been able to go to a birthday party. We worked hard to mature his sensory system through lots of chances to move through space and get his hands dirty (so to speak). He made great progress and did it quickly because mom stepped right in to helping to create a sensory lifestyle for him at home. She told me "I just had to get used to my house not always looking so neat and organized." I can't begin to tell you how happy that makes my heart feel to hear that.

WORKING SENSORY INPUT IN TO AN ALREADY BUSY DAY

I want to give you some ideas of how my family has made it a part of our lifestyle to work sensory input into our busy days, how other parents have worked it into theirs, and how you can work it into yours. These strategies can be used whether you have "typically developing" children or children with a diagnosis that involves the sensory system. Every parent, teacher, and caregiver needs a big bag of tricks!

- Prior to school, pick five activities and do each one for a minute or so. A great way to go about doing this is to have pictures of all of the sensory activities that are available to the children in your home or have them written down if the children can read. The night before, allow the children to pick five activities to be done the next morning, just as they pick out their clothes for the next day. Doing this allows children to feel in control, and they will tend to pick the activities they know are going to feel the best to them.
  - Have them crabwalk, bear walk, or wheelbarrow on the way to brush their teeth.
  - Let them use a straw at breakfast to drink the milk out of their cereal or drink their yogurt or applesauce.
  - Have them spin (sitting on a spinning office chair or by playing "helicopter") before leaving for school or while standing at the bus stop (since the bus can sometimes be an incredibly overstimulating and stressful time for a child).
  - Have them lie down on their stomach and then give them deep pressure by firmly rolling a rubber ball down their back and down the backs of their arms and legs. If you are a parent who still has to go in and wake your children up in the morning, you can do this before they even get out of bed.
  - If you wake your children up in the morning, do so with a foam paintbrush or surgical scrub brush in your hand and do the brushing techniques listed in chapter 25.
  - Have them do the tummy roll on an exercise ball or large beach ball or just have the ball out so they can bounce on it. Allow them to sit on it while they eat their breakfast.
  - Have them do some jumping jacks or spend time jumping on an indoor trampoline if you have one.
  - Choose breakfast foods wisely—perhaps chewy or crunchy foods at breakfast to increase their level of alertness and

improve neurological organization. Examples would be apple slices, a bagel, dried fruit, a granola bar, or dry cereal.
- Turn on either upbeat music or soft and calming music for auditory input while your children get dressed and eat breakfast.
- Give deep hugs when they wake up, on the way out of the door, and whenever else you can squeeze it in the day.

- After school, allow the children to run, climb, swing, etc. for at least a short period before settling down to do homework. After this playtime, use a few strategies to neurologically organize them before doing homework. For example, give them a crunchy or chewy snack, rock them side to side on a large exercise ball, then have them dig through a rice bowl or do some heavy work or proprioceptive activities. Also, let them sip on a drink through a straw while doing homework.
- Infuse homework time with sensory activities such as activities on a ball, scooter board, or jumping activities. If it is required of children that they sit still for an activity, then let them take quick breaks to do jumping jacks, crabwalk to the bathroom for a bathroom break, or stand up and play helicopter. Children will then neurologically reorganize themselves and be ready to sit back down and focus. For example, when my son needed to learn our phone number, I wrote each number on a separate sticky note and stuck it to the floor. I had him jump on the numbers in the order of our phone number. He not only learned the number, but he remembered it for the first time in the year that we had been working on it. Another example of how we do things in our house is that when my son is staring into space not focusing on his homework, we get out of our chairs and do some jumping jacks followed by spinning, then sit back down. Voila! He is now ready to focus on his work.
- Limit video games and TV. Children do not get any good sensory input during these activities, and it prohibits them from doing things that will.
- Before bed, especially if your children have a hard time sleeping, do some calming strategies such as rocking, giving deep pressure to their back and the backs of their arms and legs by firmly rolling a ball along them, scratching their backs, listen to calming music with dim lights,

rock them side to side while they are lying on their stomachs on a large therapy ball, use the brushing technique or use a foam paintbrush to "paint them," and do some deep breathing exercises.
- Try setting up different stations in each room of your house. Perhaps leave the exercise ball in one room for them to bounce and roll on. Put a small trampoline in front of the TV so they can jump while watching TV. Put a spin board or spinning chair where children can easily access it. Have a tunnel in one room for children to crawl. Leave a pillowcase out for impromptu sack races. Always provide straws for drinking through and choose meal and snack foods wisely to provide calming, alerting, or organizing input based on what your children need. When you are walking through a parking lot, allow the children to walk on the curbs for balance. Have "can steppers" set out for children to play with, etc. Have a balance cushion or balance board in the kitchen so that while you are cooking dinner of packing lunches they can stand and balance while telling you about their day. Have a rice bowl handy for them to pull out and play with while you get dinner ready (I will tell you that my kids constantly ask to get the rice bowl out. I find that it helps to calm them both.). Have putty sitting on the table for them to play with to build hand strength but also release their frustration on by mashing and stretching. Rotate objects and activities around so there is always something novel there to keep them interested.
- In the heat of the moment when you know children are about to have a meltdown or tantrum, have them start doing jumping jacks or start spinning or break out in to a crabwalk. Honestly, you can spend 20 minutes trying to calm, distract, reason, etc. with children or you can spend 30-60 seconds neurologically reorganizing them when they have obviously reached their threshold by doing a proprioceptive, vestibular, or tactile activity. We have a couch cushion in our house that my children are allowed to take off the couch and jump on while it is on the floor. We use that to jump on or a chair in our family room to spin on when things are hitting the fan in our house.
- Try to keep your children from getting overscheduled and bogged down with too many extracurricular activities. This is important so that they can come home from school and swing, run, ride bikes, shoot hoops, climb trees, hand upside down from monkey bars,

- skateboard, jump rope, pogo stick, get their hands dirty playing outside, and so on.
- Make sure that on rainy days when your children do not get the opportunity to get outside to play that you set activities up inside of your house that they can do to get sensory input. Some examples of how to do this are to let them have cotton ball races (blowing cotton balls through a straw), do scooter board activities, pull each other around while one is seated on a blanket, or play jumping games such as sack races, etc. I like to set up obstacle courses with my children incorporating several different vestibular, tactile, and proprioceptive activities on rainy days.
- Make bath or shower time a time to get sensory input with shaving cream, bathtub paints, foam soap, etc. that kids can smear all over the shower or tub with their hands. When they are done (and if they are still little enough), spend extra time drying them off and applying lotion to give them extra tactile input.
- For those of you that are teachers, encourage your students to take movement breaks throughout the day to increase their ability to focus and attend. Parents, encourage your children's teachers to allow for movement breaks to help neurologically organize their class. The few seconds to minutes spent on this will be of great benefit to each student (Which we all know will have a great benefit to the teacher as well.).
- Most of all, don't be afraid to let your children get their hands dirty, make a mess, move and explore with their hands and bodies. Obviously, you have to use your common sense, but sometimes I feel we forget to let our kids just be kids.

Let me give you some more specifics of how this all looks in my house. I have mentioned my son and the hit that his building blocks had taken during his kindergarten year. I have probably made it pretty clear that he, like just about every other child or grown-up I have ever met, has his share of sensory quirks.

My son is what I call a "doo-tee-doer." He constantly seems to be in outer space during mealtime, homework time, or when it is time to get dressed for school. Thank goodness we are starting to overcome this as he enters the teenage years but when he was in elementary school I was in full OT mode to help him focus on what he needed to be doing. I would have him get up and do J-R-C. J means jump, R means to raise your hands, and C means clap. I would say something like J-R-R-C, and he had to do those four things in order to remember what they stood for. I would do this several times changing up the order and the number of motor commands I linked together to be done at one time. After that, I would have him spin 10 times. Or I would have him do some kind of jumping activity or just plain old jumping jacks. We would play a quick game of Simon Says to neurologically organize him so he could then sit and focus. Worked like a charm. If I did one of these activities prior to sending him upstairs to get dressed, make his bed, and brush his teeth, he magically could get them all done without forgetting any steps. If I didn't do one of these activities prior to sending him upstairs, without fail, he would forget at least one of the steps in this process (even though he had had to do the same four things every morning for a few years).

When he was in a state of melt-down and there was nothing we could do to reason with him, I would throw out, "let's spin" or "let's have a crab walk race." We would do one of those activities, then I would have him lie down on his tummy while I firmly rubbed down his back and the backs of his arms and legs with a rubber ball. Another great tip that worked like a charm was to have him start listing something verbally (food he likes, friends' names, restaurants he likes to eat at, etc.). Crisis averted. Temper tantrum diffused. I got my son back without losing my temper and my mind along with it.

One afternoon, he came home from school, and after his sister looked at him the wrong way, he had a complete emotional meltdown. I knew at this point that he had had a long day and needed a boost to help him self-organize his emotions. I kept going down my list of tricks, and he wanted nothing to do with any of them. At this point, I gave him a few minutes to be alone with his tears, then sat at the kitchen table with my dry rice bowl (See tactile activities in chapter 25.) and therapy putty which is basically play-do on steroids. Therapy putty is great for proprioceptive input because of how tough it is to manipulate and the resistance it provides. He gradually came over to me at the table and his tears were soon forgotten. He got lost in the rice bowl as he started running his hands through it feeling the soft texture of it on his skin. We then took turns hiding pennies in the therapy putty for the other person to find. He had to use a lot of strength for this and got a lot of great sensory input through the resistance that it provided to his muscles. We did this for a while, and he was like a new kid. No more tears. No more meltdown, just a good boost to the sensory system which helped him to reorganize his brain during this time of mass disorganization.

My son also had a hard time memorizing things such as our address, phone number, or his birthday. As soon as I would have him jump it out (For example, I write the digits of our phone number on separate pieces of sticky paper and have him jump on each number.) or recite them after we had done our spinning, a miracle happened. Not only did he remember them, but he had learned them for good.

This is the same boy who walked in circles while he told me stories (and still does to this day). I realized he was giving himself vestibular input to help him focus so he could concentrate while telling me the story. Because I knew this, I would set up vestibular activities all over our house and, without fail, he always gravitated toward them. He had a mini trampoline on which he jumped while watching TV or playing WII. He had a balance board in his playroom to stand on while he does other activities. He would bounce and roll all day all over our big exercise ball, and would swing for hours when able. Since I realized what he was seeking, I could set things up so he could get the sensory input he was craving all day long and whenever he needed it. He is a "typically developing" child, but, boy, what a boost he was getting to his sensory foundation. The best part about this is that it doesn't take much of my time or money. When I would spin him on our swivel chair in our family room or stop to do an activity with him, he didn't understand fully why I was doing these things, but he loved it. He was getting my attention and having fun doing it and sometimes that goes farther than anything else! Now that he is 13-years-old we don't have to do as much of this, but there are days we still have to put the wheels in motion.

Let me give you one more little trick that I like to use and think it important. It is a great idea to keep these activities fresh by rotating them around. I would leave one or two fine motor activities or sensory activities that they could do with their hands on our kitchen table. I would put the therapy putty on the table for a day or two. Then I would put that away and put the rice bowl out for a few days. Next, came the pop beads or Lite Brite for fine motor work. Then it was pipe cleaners and beads for more fine motor work and then good old crayons, scissors, glue, and construction paper so they could use their imaginations and draw. By keeping new things constantly popping up for your children to do, it keeps the excitement alive (and they don't get bored so easily).

The other thing I did a lot was to rotate some of my gross motor things around and put them out where the kids will literally trip over them so they are more prone to stop and play with them if even just for a minute. For example, when my kids hadn't used the trampoline for a while, I would set it out right in the middle of the foyer so they would stop and jump every time they walked by it. After a day or two of this, I would put the scooter board in its place. Next thing you know my kids were wheeling themselves and each other around on it. After a few days of this, I would put the balance cushion or balance board out for them to stand on. I liked to put this in a doorway with a ball suspended from a string for them to hit back and forth (a great visual activity). When they were watching TV, I would tiptoe in and put the exercise ball in front of the TV and next thing I know they were bouncing on it while watching TV. I would also do this with "can steppers", the spin board, and wobble deck. What you see is that I was not necessarily having to do these things with them, I just made them accessible and kept them fresh and exciting so they would be drawn to doing them without my having to urge them to do so.

My kids have come a long way so we don't have to do nearly the amount of sensory activities we used to have to do but it's still important. You may think I'm crazy, but we have indoor riding toys. We have a ripstik and hover board that are only allowed in the house (once the wheels have been marked up by the sidewalk, they are no longer allowed in the house). My kids will ride for hours (Truly . . . hours!) on these toys in our house. I have even let them rollerblade in the house out of desperation. On rainy days, we have set up obstacle courses in the garage using cones or ice chests as the obstacles and they maneuver around them on their riding toys. They still love the putty and rice bowl and it's still a great after school transition activity. My daughter reads hanging upside down over the edge of the couch or her bed or spins in a chair. She also loves cooking and getting her hands dirty baking. I have swivel stools at my kitchen table so they can spin while they eat and get the movement they need. They are at an age where electronics become a much bigger fight so we have strict boundaries and make sure we have lots of outdoor activities planned. As I'm writing, my eleven-year-old daughter is standing next to me watching GoNoodle videos. This is a great resource for videos that make movement lots of fun and is a great thing to do before school or homework or any other time you need a quick and fun movement break.

I was speaking to a group of moms the other day and a mom jokingly said, "I guess I need to redecorate my house." Well, yes and no. You don't have to redecorate necessarily, but you do need to think of ways that you can make it part of your children's lifestyle for them to get sensory input. This means that the things that will give them this great sensory input have to be readily available to them and has to catch their interest. These strategies aren't hard. They just take a little thought and putting the right things in place.

> Don't forget, either, that there is NO BETTER WAY for your children to get great sensory input than by letting them run outside, climb, jump, swing, and explore with their hands outside during free play.

Hopefully, what you see is that it isn't hard or time-consuming to use some of these strategies once you get some of the necessary tools in place. If you provide opportunities for sensory input, children will often take to them without much cueing or prompting. Don't forget, either, that there is no better way for your children to get great sensory input than by letting them run outside, climb, jump, swing, and explore with their hands outside during free play.

REMEMBER: You have to LEARN TO MOVE and MOVE TO LEARN!

CHAPTER 23

PROPRIOCEPTIVE ACTIVITIES

Proprioceptive activities are activities that allow children to use their muscles and joints. The more resistance the activities provide to the children's muscles or the more load they allow the child to bear through the joints, the better.

- **Jumping or hopping activities** - This includes trampolines, bounce houses, jumping jacks, hopscotch, sack races, jumping on one leg, or jumping up to touch a target such as letters on a wall to form spelling words.
- **Heavy work** - This includes pushing, pulling, lifting, or carrying heavy objects. Example - pulling a wagon full of rocks, pushing or carrying or a heavy box or laundry basket, carrying a heavy stack of books, tug of war, or pushing a vacuum cleaner. Having your kids help you with housework or yard work is a win-win!
- **Deep pressure activities -** Deep pressure can be both calming and neurologically organizing (meaning that it helps children to get mentally prepared and ready to focus). Deep pressure activities include bear hugs, applying deep pressure by rolling a ball down their backs and the backs of their arms and legs, and massages to their muscles (especially the feet).
- **Deep pressure items** - This includes weighted blankets, vests, lap pads, or caps (you can Google these items to get information on how to order).
- Crab walking, bear walking, and wheelbarrow racing
- **Activities on the floor while on their hands and knees** - This includes doing puzzles, drawing with sidewalk chalk on the driveway, or playing a board game.
- **Climbing** - This includes climbing on playground equipment or any other safe climbing activity.
- **Bouncing** - This includes bouncing on such things as a hippity-hop ball or while sitting on a large exercise ball.

- **Exercise** - This includes things such as push-ups, pull-ups, planks, holding "superman", using weights or exercise bands, burpees running, lunges, etc.
- **Activities on the floor lying on their stomach and propped on their elbows** - This is a great position to be in while coloring, doing homework, or reading.
- **Chewy or crunchy foods** - We receive a great deal of proprioceptive input through our jaw muscles as we chew. Some healthy examples are: dried fruit, beef jerky, fruit leathers, bagels, granola bars (especially with caramel), cheese, celery or carrot sticks, apple slices, fruit gummies, pretzels, nuts, popcorn, dry cereal, toast, dried veggie or fruit chips, rice cakes, and pita chips.
- **Drinking through a straw** - Drinking through a straw also gives good proprioceptive input to our oral musculature. You can do applesauce, yogurt, and shakes through a straw in addition to your normal liquids. Drinking out of a water bottle with a straw during the school day is another good trick.

Pinterest is a great resource for other fun proprioceptive activities.

Don't forget that it is important to work these activities in throughout your children's day and make proprioceptive input a part of your children's lifestyle. An important thing to remember, as well, is that **when all else fails, give your children proprioceptive input**. This input is rarely overstimulating and can be calming, help counter hypersensitivities in the other sensory systems, and neurologically organizing. It can also help increase children's level of alertness, ability to focus, and decrease anxiety.

CHAPTER 24

VESTIBULAR ACTIVITIES

Activities that involve moving the head in circular, side to side, or angular (think about leaning down then up) patterns, are great ways to give vestibular input. Here are some suggestions on ways you can encourage your child to do just that:

- **Spinning** - This can be done on a sit and spin, spin disk, office chair or any other swivel chair, on a swing or tire swing, or standing up with arms out to the sides playing "helicopter." Just be careful not to overdo it as this can make some children feel sick or can have other adverse effects on them.
- **Rolling** - Log rolling across the floor, rolling down a hill, somersaults
- **Scooter board** - (order online) Children can propel themselves forward, backward, sideways, or in circles on the board or they can hold on to a dowel or long stick while someone pulls them.
- **Exercise ball** - Activities done while children lie on their stomachs on a large exercise ball and move forward and backward and side to side.
- **Rocking** - You can hold your children firmly and rock them rhythmically side to side or forward and backward if you don't have a chair that rocks. Children also enjoy laying on their stomachs on a large exercise ball while you slowly and rhythmically rock them forward and backward or side to side.
- **Balance activities** - These can be done while standing on one leg, on a balance board, balance cushion, BOSU ball, a street curb, balance beam or 2x4's, etc.
- **Being upside down** - This can be hanging from playground equipment, hanging upside down over the edge of furniture or on an exercise ball.
- **Playground equipment** - This includes swings, teeter-totters, merry-go-rounds

- **Can Steppers** - (order online) These are great for balance and body awareness.
- **Gross motor activities** - This includes playing catch, kicking a ball playing basketball, tag, or hopscotch.

Pinterest is a great resource for lots of fun vestibular activities.

As with all sensory input, remember that it is important to build these activities into your children's day and make opportunities for them to receive vestibular input as part of their lifestyle.

If you have children who are fearful of movement, start small. Never force them in to doing anything that increases their fears or anxieties and watch for dizziness or loss of balance during activities. If your children are fearful of spinning, start with less aversive activities like gentle rocking, balancing activities, toe touches, over-under, or windmill. Work your way up to spinning by letting them play "helicopter" and spin in circles a few times while standing or play "Ring Around the Rosey." If swinging causes your child to be fearful, start by swinging with them while they are seated on your lap. Only have your children do as much as they can tolerate.

Some children are aversive to one type of vestibular activity but not another. For example, some children can swing all day but if they spin in a circle they get extremely dizzy. If this is the case, have them do the type of vestibular input they can tolerate and you can gradually try to build up their tolerance to other forms of vestibular input. Just remember to let the children be the guide on this one.

Another thing to monitor is whether or not your children become over-aroused by vestibular input. Vestibular input can be overstimulating for some children and overwhelm them. If this is the case, you may want to make sure your children focus on proprioceptive (or heavy work input) and making sure to use this type of input after vestibular input. If your children tend to over do it with vestibular input because of the enjoyment they get from it, but you know that it will cause them to become disorganized or overstimulated, then you may need to monitor them closely with this. Vestibular and proprioceptive input can both be neurologically organizing; however, vestibular input can be overstimulating while proprioceptive input is calming. "More is better" is not always the case with vestibular input; however, it is very important that children get it (just within their limits of what they can tolerate).

CHAPTER 25

TACTILE ACTIVITIES

Kids who crave extra touch, or seem to have a tactile hunger, need opportunities for extra touch input during their day. They need it in order to self-organize, self-regulate, focus, etc. Believe it or not, kids who are sensitive to or have trouble with touch input need opportunities to receive it, as well. In fact, it is very important that they get it. These kids need opportunities to experience different kinds of touch in order to build a properly functioning foundation that will allow them to interpret the tactile world around them properly.

- **Brushing** – You can order surgical scrub brushes on amazon. I recommend the scrub brush but you can also use a foam paintbrush that you can get for less than $1.00 in the paint supply section at your local big-box home improvement store. When brushing, use firm pressure (hard enough to move the skin) and slow, steady strokes. You can brush over clothing if needed but direct contact on skin is preferred. Just be consistent and do not move from skin to over clothing.
    - Brush the arms (covering as much surface area as possible) five strokes in an up and down motion, covering the area twice
    - Brush the palms of their hands five times.
    - Brush their back five times up and down and then five times side to side
    - Brush their other arm
    - Brush the legs below the knee covering as much surface area as possible five strokes up and down two times.
    - Brush the feet holding one hand on top of the foot. Move the brush in a sweeping motion moving the top hand in sync with the brushing hand five times

  For a child who is extremely tactile defensive, you may need to start with few strokes and build up their tolerance. Starting with the deep pressure techniques mentioned in chapter 23 will help to prepare the tactile defensive child for this brushing. I recommend you always have a brush handy and do this frequently you can do this as often as every 1 ½-2 hours. Follow this up by having your child do some jumping activities (jumping jacks work great). This will give them joint compressions (proprioceptive input) after the tactile input which will help to enhance the benefits. You may not notice instant benefits from this, but if you do this brushing technique consistently over the course of 2 weeks, you will start to see some improvements. Please refer to https://sensoryprocessingdisorderparentsupport.com/wilbarger-brushingcompressions.php for more details on the brushing protocol.

- **Rice bowl activities** – Fill a large bowl with dry rice and put hidden treasure in it for which children can dig. You can also use other textures to fill the bowl such as dry beans or noodles.
- **Playing in foam soap or shaving cream** – Children can do this in the shower or squirt it on a cookie sheet and have fun. They can use this activity while doing spelling words or any other learning activity. They can write the answers in foam soap.
- **Bathtub paint** – They can paint while taking a bath and make it fun.
- **Playing with toys** – Toys with texture or tactile qualities (such as squishy balls, spikey balls, soft blankets, etc.) provide a calming effect for children with these deficiencies.
- **Lying in a tactile box** – Fill a large box (Appliance boxes work great.) with stuffed animals, sponges, foam pieces, soft blankets, etc. and have children lie in it.
- **Playing in sandbox** – This can be a fun activity and at the same time provide the stimulation needed.
- **Fidget box or bag** – Make a box or a bag to keep with you on the go or for your children to have in their classroom filled with objects with different tactile qualities that are pleasing to them. These objects may be bumpy, rough, soft, squishy, textured, smooth, etc. Some examples are a squishy ball, small balls filled with sand for resistance when squeezing, soft stuffed animals, etc. This is a great trick to use in the classroom with the teacher's permission to allow children to get extra

input to "fill their cup" during the school day so that they can focus on their work.

- **Deep pressure** – Deep pressure is a proprioceptive activity (refer to chapter 23) but I want to mention it here because it is calming as it can override the "fright, flight, or fight" response that children with tactile sensitivity may exhibit. Therefore, deep pressure is great to use prior to, during, and after an activity that you know may spark a negative reaction by your child. Some instances where deep pressure may come in handy are prior to your children having to walk on the beach or in the grass or put shoes and socks on.

  Deep pressure can be done and used in many different ways but should always be done lovingly. I always resort to deep pressure when children are in a very heightened state of arousal (i.e., having a tantrum or fit, or when they are worked up or seem overstimulated, etc.). Deep bear hugs, deep muscle massages, foot massages, pressure down through the shoulders, and firmly rubbing a rubber ball down their back while they are lying on their stomachs, are all examples of deep pressure.

Again, Pinterest is a great resource full of fun and creative tactile activities.

I mentioned that even children who have a tactile defensiveness will benefit from tactile input. As with anything, however, don't force it. Ease your children into it and allow them to explore and get comfortable with certain textures before moving on to something else. For example, most kids really love the dry rice bowl. Let your children get really comfortable with playing with that and let them do so for a week or two before moving on to shave cream or foam soap. If this is going to be scary for them, let them use a foam paintbrush first for this activity and then progress toward letting them use their hands for it. Give them lots of back scratches or rubs (skin on skin) for a while to expose them to a tactile sensation. Do the brushing frequently as this is often perceived as harmless and quite pleasurable to most children. Do these activities for a while building up to the tactile box, sandbox, or tactile tunnel. Always remember to use deep pressure prior to and after exposing children to a texture that may be frightening to them.

CHAPTER 26

STRATEGIES TO USE WITH CHILDREN WHO ARE SENSORY UNDER-SENSITIVE

In chapters 23, 24, and 25 there are specific ideas for activities to use with children to build their proprioceptive, vestibular, and tactile foundations. With children who have SUR, you want to provide lots of opportunities for them to get these specific types of sensory input. To fill their cup, they need fast and intense input and lots of it. These kids do not need to be sitting on the couch or playing video games. They need to be moving. I tell kids that for every hour they spend watching TV or playing video games, they need to spend two hours running, climbing, jumping, riding bikes, etc. Here are some basic strategies of intervention to use with children who have SUR:

- **Use fast and intense sensory input** – You obviously have to use your common sense on this one and make sure you provide supervision. What I mean by this is offer activities that will provide several sensory inputs at the same time, that will use more muscle groups or give a greater amount of input, and change things up frequently. For example, to give several sensory inputs at the same time have your children play in the rice bowl while listening to loud music, or have them stand on a balance board or balance cushion while hitting a suspended ball back and forth, or have them lay on the scooter board on their stomach moving in a linear fashion while using the heavy work muscles of their arms to advance themselves forward on it.

    To change things up frequently, I like to do obstacle courses. I like to have children do something like ride on the scooter board, then jump on the trampoline, then balance on the balance beam or 2x4's, then run across the room holding a medicine ball, then crabwalk to the finish line. Be creative with this but use several activities that provide proprioceptive and vestibular input and have them go from one activity right into the next.

STRATEGIES TO USE WITH CHILDREN WHO ARE SENSORY UNDER-SENSITIVE

Activities that provide more intense input are those such as spinning for intense vestibular input, jumping, crab walking, or wheelbarrow racing for proprioceptive input (think heavy work that involves lots of muscles), and rougher, pokier, squishier textures for tactile input.

- **Provide them with lots and lots of opportunities for enhanced sensory input** – You will sometimes notice that under-sensitive children will spend more time in front of the TV or playing video games; they may prefer more sedentary activities such as these. Limit this but make sure that even when doing sedentary activities they are getting sensory input. Let them sit on an exercise ball if playing a handheld video game, have them jump on a mini indoor trampoline while watching TV, let them sit on a balance cushion, exercise ball, or kneel while eating meals or doing homework, let them do their reading while lying on their stomachs on an exercise ball, or keep a rice bowl or therapy putty handy for them to sit and manipulate with their hands.

- **Find activities that are meaningful and motivating to your children** – Obviously, if the activity means nothing to them, then they won't want to do it. Know what your children are interested in and then design activities to incorporate that. For instance, if your children like puzzles, have them lay on their stomach on an exercise ball while doing puzzles. If your children love Angry Birds, set up an obstacle course where they are the "angry bird" moving through space on a scooter board to go and knock down a stack of cones or empty milk jugs. If your children like to play games, play Twister, Elefun, charades or any other game that requires movement. Catch my drift?

Here is a list of a few more ideas that you can use to work this in to your children's day:

- Work jumping into their daily activities, especially learning activities. Let them work on flashcards for math or spelling or facts for a test while jumping on a trampoline. Have them jump on to the flashcard that has the right answer. Have the answers posted on cards high enough up on the wall that they have to jump up to touch the right answer or the next letter when spelling a word.
- Have them crabwalk or wheelbarrow at transition times (from one room to the next, to go brush their teeth before school, when they are going to use the restroom, etc.).

- When you see them starting to drift away either at home or in the classroom, have them stand up and do jumping jacks or spin in circles.
- Before they need to be able to sit and focus, let them play outside for a while.
- Do J-R-C where you say the letter and they have to jump, raise their hands, or clap according to the letters you spoke. Make it more difficult by giving them the command of J-R-J-R-C or C-R-R-C-J and so on.
- Keep an exercise ball, trampoline, or balance board in different rooms where your children spend a lot of time and encourage them to use them often. Let them jump while they are watching TV, balance while they stand to eat a meal, snack, or do their homework, or sit on the exercise ball to perform these activities.
- Pull them around on the scooter board or keep the board lying around so the children will push each other around. When pulling them, do it fast, changing directions often.
- Let them keep a fidget tool in their pocket. Find something they can fidget with using their hands inconspicuously throughout the day when they are feeling antsy.
- Spread foaming hand soap on a cookie sheet and have them practice writing spelling words, math problems, history facts (dates, people, places, etc) on it to get extra tactile input while learning.

These activities are not hard and do not require fancy tools or equipment or a lot of time. Work them in as often as you can. Have children start their day with a few of these activities to get their cup full before they are expected to start performing whether at home or school. Have a list and let your child pick a few activities to do before school, after school, before and during homework, before a sporting event, family gathering, trip to the store, etc.

> GOAL: Provide your children with a "JUST RIGHT" challenge; one that will be motivating and stimulate their sensory system but not over stimulate them.

Goal: Provide your children with a "just right" challenge; one that will be motivating and stimulate their sensory system but not over stimulate them.

CHAPTER 27

STRATEGIES TO USE WITH CHILDREN WHO ARE SENSORY OVER-SENSITIVE

The strategies we use for children who are over responsive focus on helping them reach a normal arousal level. It is important to teach your children about what gets them into a state of overarousal so that they can learn how to self-regulate. It is also important to use strategies that will help to calm their sensory system and organize them neurologically. Once this happens, they will be able to better tolerate the stimuli that they are aversive to.

Refer back to chapters 23, 24, and 25 for proprioceptive, vestibular, and tactile activities and to chapter 29 for a list of calming and self-regulation strategies to help make sense of some of the following and for further ideas. Some specific strategies used for children with SOR include the following:

- **Provide calming input to help with their level of arousal** – If your children are over-sensitive to sensory input then more than likely they will be in a state of overarousal. When this is the case, you need to help normalize their level of arousal and reach a calmer and more balanced state. To do this, provide slow, rhythmical, quiet activities for them such as massage, deep pressure, or back rubs (you can use the ball roll talked about in chapter 23).
- **Provide opportunities for heavy work** – Heavy work provides proprioceptive input which is believed to help with calming and neurologically organizing children. It is provided by pushing, pulling, or carrying weighted objects. It can also be provided through deep pressure input to the joints. Refer to chapter 23 for a list of proprioceptive activities but here are some examples of activities that require heavy work:
    - Pushing or carrying a heavy laundry basket
    - Carrying a heavy stack of books from the classroom to the library

- Pulling a wagon with another child or something heavy in it
- Providing heavy work opportunities within children's natural context (home, school, etc.) such as vacuuming or carrying grocery bags in the house
- Giving bear hugs
- Pushing into the wall
- Holding your hands up so your children can push in to your hands as hard as they can
- Doing push-ups
- Squeezing therapy putty (order on amazon) or Crazy Aaron's Thinking Putty
- Sitting in bean bag chairs (due to the fact that they envelop you when you sit in them)

- **Provide vestibular activities that are calming such as rocking and swinging.** To rock them, try holding the children in your arms and provide pressure as firmly as they can tolerate. Slowly and rhythmically rock back and forth with them in your arms. You can also have them lie on a large therapy ball and you hold on to them and rock them side to side or forward and backward slowly. For swinging activities, have your children swing in a slow, forward and backward motion (as they tolerate).
- **Provide a "time in" spot** – This is not "time out" but instead "time in." They are not punished but, instead, are spending some time by themselves to regroup and decompress. Have them fill their "time in" spot with things that are comforting to them such as a bean bag chair, soft blankets or stuffed animals, objects to squeeze or manipulate with their hands. Set this spot up with low lighting and make sure that your children can be in their "time in" spot without interruption.
- **Have sensory activities or objects around your house and readily available to your children** – This will allow your children to get sensory input when they are ready and as they feel the need. In our house, I have sensory things such as therapy putty, a dry rice bowl, a scooter board, a balance cushion, an indoor trampoline, a spin board, a large exercise ball, etc. accessible to my kids. When my son was younger and was over-aroused or seemed disorganized, he would often ask for the dry rice bowl or the therapy putty. I would sporadically put certain things like the scooter board or trampoline in

STRATEGIES TO USE WITH CHILDREN WHO ARE SENSORY OVER-SENSITIVE

the middle of the foyer so the kids felt the urge to use them every time they walked by them. I still put the spin board and exercise ball in front of the TV and the balance cushion in the kitchen. Keeping them out and in their line of sight makes them more apt to use them as they feel the urge.

- **Slowly expose your children to the sensory stimuli to which they are sensitive** – While avoiding the sensory stimuli that get your children over-aroused can be beneficial at times, it is important that they are exposed to it so that they can learn to become more comfortable with the stimuli. Exposing your children to sensory stimulation in increments can be better than completely avoiding the stimulation. For example, it may be best to avoid an amusement park if your child has vestibular oversensitivity. However, exposing your child slowly to vestibular input is important. You can start with some simple windmills, slow swinging, or playing helicopter. Increase the intensity, frequency, and duration as your children's tolerance builds. If they are afraid of swinging, start by having them sit on your lap and just sitting on the swing, then swing slowly with them on your lap, then let them sit on the swing by themselves, then let them start swinging slowly at their comfort level.

- **Provide chewy snacks or opportunities for your children to suck** – This allows them to use the heavy muscles of their mouths which provides proprioceptive input for calming. Some good choices are chewing granola bars, fruit leathers, bubble gum, drinking applesauce, pudding, or milkshakes through a straw, etc.

- **Provide predictability** – Make sure they have plenty of notice if you are going to make changes to their surroundings, schedules, etc. Picture schedules work great. I like to have pictures of the days' activities for these children. If something is going to change, let them swap out the picture of the event, thus helping them to feel more in control of the situation. If pictures are not available then we will write out a schedule and continuously refer back to it so the children know what comes next. If we have to make changes to the schedule then we make the changes on our written schedule. When out in public, make sure you have your "sensory bag" ready (see chapter 29) and lots of games or activities up your sleeve that your children are familiar with to help prevent a state of overarousal or help to calm them if they reach a state of overarousal.

> **GOAL:** Provide your children with a "JUST RIGHT" challenge; one that will be motivating and stimulate their sensory system but not over stimulate them.

The trick is to pay attention to what works and what doesn't work for your children. Ask them how certain activities that you use help them feel. Take note of this. If they liked it, it's a keeper; it means that it works for them. If they don't, toss it.

Goal: Provide your children with a "just right" challenge; one that will be motivating and stimulate their sensory system but not over stimulate them.

CHAPTER 28

ADD/ADHD ACTIVITIES

Oftentimes children with ADD and ADHD are seeking out movement and seem disorganized and distractible because they are not at their optimum level of arousal. Remember, that a large percentage of children with ADD and ADHD are also thought to have sensory processing difficulties and many of them are craving more sensory input. It is important for you to use this book to help you determine the state of their sensory cups and learn which cups they are working to fill, or which cups may be overflowing.

Keep in mind that children can't sit still until they know how to move. Also, keep in mind that kids have to move to learn and move to learn. Knowing that many children with ADD and ADHD are seeking out more sensory input in order to get to an optimum level of arousal means that we need to give these children opportunities to move and opportunities to fill their cup when needed. To do this, refer back to chapter 26 for a list of activities that will help to do just that. Also, refer back to chapters 23, 24, and 25 for a list of proprioceptive, vestibular, and tactile activities to fill their day with.

Make sure that these children have movement breaks built in to learning and homework time and you may have to think outside of the box and offer other alternatives to having to sit still while doing work. For example, let them sit on an exercise ball or balance cushion, let them kneel on a chair with one leg while standing on the other, or let them turn their chairs sideways eliminating the ability to rest their back against the back of the chair which allows for movement. Working with your children's teachers so that together you can find ways to help them reach their optimum level of arousal so they can focus is crucial.

For children who are seeking out sensory input, focus on proprioceptive and vestibular activities and the strategies that we use with children who are sensory under-sensitive. Use these activities at the start of their day before they go to school, camp, daycare, ball games, play dates, etc. Then use them again after school, before dinner, during the school day (when permitted by the teacher), and any other time during the day when you can tell the children are struggling with their arousal level. Remember that proprioceptive input can be calming and neurologically organizing. So, when all else fails, give proprioceptive input and lots of it. Give your children lots of opportunities to use their large muscles, do resisted activities, and do heavy work. Make sure the time these children spend on video games is kept to a minimum and the time they spend riding bikes, climbing, swinging, jumping, exploring their environment through touch, and time to use their large muscles is a priority for each and every day.

> GIVE YOUR CHILDREN lots of opportunities to use their large muscles, do resisted activities, and do heavy work.

Give these strategies two to three months of wholehearted efforts making sure your children have some sort of tactile, vestibular, and proprioceptive input throughout their day. Work with their teacher, if needed, to use the suggested solutions for the classroom or come up with other ways that may work for your children to give them the sensory input they are longing for in the classroom. When you use these strategies, you will be surprised and amazed when you realize not only what you are seeing but also the behaviors that you are no longer seeing! You may realize medication is still needed but don't stop providing the sensory stimuli as you now know that a majority of kids with ADD and ADHD also have sensory integration dysfunction. Remember, our brains have neuroplasticity and can make changes when given the tools to do so.

CHAPTER 29

SELF-REGULATION/CALMING ACTIVITIES

Below is a list of activities and strategies to use with your children who need help to self-regulate. Remember that we all have to learn to self-regulate, it's just that some of our children require more help to do so.

1. A key in helping your children learn to self-regulate or control their emotions and behaviors is **to help them identify their emotions**. Talk about them with your children. This may be easier to do after the fact or after the storm has settled, but it is important to help them put a name to the emotion they were just or are currently experiencing. Sad, happy, nervous, anxious, mad, angry, excited, overwhelmed, etc. You can role-play these feelings, take turns acting out each one of these emotions, or draw a picture with the face of a person and their expressions when experiencing one of these emotions. Being able to talk to your children about how they are feeling and then talking about a self-regulation strategy to use in each of these instances will help in the future. It may take weeks, months, or even years of doing this, but it will eventually pay off and you will have children who then can independently use strategies to help control their emotions or behaviors. A great way to model this is to explain to your child your own emotions. For example:

- "Mommy is feeling very frustrated right now so I am going to go stand outside for a minute and take a deep breath."
- "This song makes me feel so happy and energetic and want to get up and dance."
- "I am feeling so tired right now. I may go splash some cold water on my face or do some exercising to help me wake up."

2. When there is an experience or situation that you know will send your children into a state of "fight, flight, or fright," **gradually work them into it**. For example, if your children don't like to swing, place them on your lap and just sit on the swing one day. The next day slowly

swing for a very short period of time with your children. Build like this until your children feel comfortable sitting on the swing themselves. If they are afraid of getting their hair cut, have them just go with you or other family members to have a haircut and have them sit to the side doing a fun activity such as coloring or playing with stickers. Work up to having them sit on your lap while you get your haircut. Do scissor activities with adult supervision so they become comfortable with scissors. Let them play "barber" and pretend to fix your hair. Take them in to meet the barber or hairdresser so that they begin to feel comfortable. Then, when you think the children are ready, let them take the plunge and get a haircut. I had a parent tell me that her child was extremely fearful of getting a shot. She said that she poked him gently with a toothpick until he got used to feeling something prick him and realized it was going to be ok and he had what it took to handle it.

3. **Prepare the children well in advance for any changes.** If you are going to change the route on the way home or change the order in which things are going to take place, talk about it. Having pictures of the tasks that make up the daily routine or having each item written down can be helpful. If something has to change, let the children change the order of the pictures or written tasks themselves. This will allow them to feel in control. Give lots of cueing such as "We are leaving the park in 10 minutes" then "We are leaving the park in 5 minutes," etc. If they are getting a new teacher, arrange a time for them to sit and talk to the teacher in advance and get familiar with them if at all possible.

4. **Be prepared for situations that you know will be overstimulating and that will upset your children.** If you know the grocery store is tough because of the bright lights and smells, have lots of fun games to play while you are in the store to help distract the children. Play "I spy" or play the letter game trying to find each letter in the alphabet as you go through the store.

5. Another way to be prepared for situations that you know will be overstimulating for your children or will bring on an inappropriate emotional response is to **have a sensory bag**. If your children crave movement and sensation or need help to maintain a level of alertness or arousal, have a backpack filled with goodies such as high bounce

SELF-REGULATION/CALMING ACTVITIES

putty, resistance balls, senso balls, light-up toys, small hand weights, Theraband, and any other little gadget that they can squeeze that will provide texture and resistance and will keep their hands busy. You can often find these types of items in the dollar section of your local big-box, dollar store, Learning Express, or a craft store such as Michael's. If your children get overstimulated easily and need calming toys, then fill a backpack with soft, plush toys, smooth toys, and familiar toys that will be comforting to them.

6. Encourage your children to take a **"time in."** This is not "time out" but instead "time in." They are not punished but just need to remove themselves from the situation for a minute to regroup. I love to utilize this strategy with my own kids. I tell them they are not being punished, but they need to spend a minute alone in their rooms to pull themselves together. This works great. A few minutes by themselves makes them new children

7. Allow them to have a **spot that is all theirs** and is set up with calming input. A corner, a room, a closet, wherever it may be. Have a bean bag chair in there, low lighting, the music that they like, their stuffed animals, anything that they have identified is calming to them. Encourage them to go to their spot when they are over-aroused or during a "time in."

8. I like to have kids **come up with a list of the things that help them to feel better** when their "head and heart feel as if they are going crazy." I help them, but they will usually come up with some great ideas. Many of them will mention lying with their stuffed animals. We will also list things like therapy putty, rice bowl, ball rubs, back rubs, "time in" in their rooms, rocking on the ball, etc. This helps them to start to self-regulate so as soon as the situation escalates you can refer to their list.

9. **Have a "bag of tricks"** that you can turn to at any time. When my children are over-aroused or upset and no amount of rationalizing is going to help the situation, I pull from my bag of tricks and the things that I know that they respond best to. It may be spinning, deep pressure rubs with the ball (refer to number 10), crab walking, wheelbarrow racing, or just a firm bear hug. Once you know what your child responds best to, make a mental note and pull those activities out when needed.

10. **Use deep pressure strategies when they are upset.** Deep pressure (or proprioceptive input) can have a calming effect. When you see your children are visibly upset, try giving them a deep bear hug lasting as long as needed. Hugs not only provide proprioceptive input but they also cause a release of oxytocin. When we are stressed out our cortisol levels rise. When we are feeling loved and bonding, oxytocin is released. Oxytocin and cortisol have a love-hate relationship as they work in opposition to each other. When one goes up, the other goes down.

    This deep pressure will help them not only feel loved and supported, but it will also give them the deep pressure that will help calm them. Another way do give them deep pressure is by simply pressing down firmly on their shoulders. A strategy I use a lot with my own kids is rolling a ball firmly down their back. I have them lie down on their stomach and I firmly roll a rubber ball up and down their backs slowly and rhythmically. It works like a charm.

11. Hold your arms up with palms facing out. **Tell the children to press as hard as they can into your hands.** This can be fun as they think they are trying to push you over (and definitely let them win); however, what is really happening is that they are getting deep pressure, which again, is calming input. They can also push against a wall with their hands as hard as they can.

12. Encourage your children to **use objects that provide resistance** such as lifting weights, pushing a laundry basket full of books down the hall, or pulling on Theratubing or Theraband when upset. This will allow them to receive heavy work input or proprioceptive input.

13. **Rock them.** If they are young enough, hold the children and rock them in a rocking chair. If you don't have a rocking chair handy, just hold them and rock back and forth rhythmically. Laying them on their stomach on a big exercise ball (preferably less than 22 inches for a smaller children and increase the size as they grow) and then rocking them slowly and rhythmically side to side or forward and backward in a slow and calm manner will typically quickly slow children down and calm them.

14. Work with children to **facilitate slow and deep breathing** having them breath in through their nose (as if smelling the birthday cake)

and out through their mouth through gently pursed lips (as if gently blowing out the birthday candles).

Let me give you a brief example of how one mom was able to think on the spot of a way to help calm her child. They were leaving a situation that she knew had her son over stimulated. They were getting in the car and she didn't know what to do at that point to help calm him down before the ride home. She looked around, didn't see anything, and then shouted, "Punch the seat!" She encouraged him to punch the back of the passenger seat to get the proprioceptive input he needed to help calm him. This same mom would allow her son to kick his exercise ball when frustrated to get that same calming proprioceptive input. I think this is a great example of a mom thinking on the spot, knowing what her child needed, and finding ways to give him what he needed to help him self-regulate (or calm himself).

The overall goal is to teach your children strategies so they will start to learn what they can do when they feel overwhelmed. Use these strategies, and always explain to them why you are using them and, over time, they will start to learn to use the strategies without your cueing them to do so. I like to ask children questions such as how a certain activity makes them feel or how they are feeling right now and what do they think they can do to help them feel better. I like to compare what is going on in their brain to a race car on a race track. I ask them if they feel like their brain is going super fast like a race car going around the race track or if their brain is feeling like it is going super slow like a race car just sitting on the race track. We then talk about what they think will help their race car to slow down or speed up. I will give them suggestions when needed but often times children can come up with some ideas that they know will help them to feel better. The key is to help them learn to determine how they are feeling and what is going to help them. You may find a few strategies work best. Focus on those and then work with the children to help them learn to self-regulate in the future.

CONCLUSION

I hope that you have a better understanding now of why you may see certain behaviors in your children, as well as the connection between their behavior and their sensory system. I also hope you understand how important a strong and firm sensory foundation is for just about everything our children do whether they have a diagnosis or not. More than anything, I hope that you feel empowered in knowing what you can do to help. Children will show us what they need. It is our job to find acceptable and appropriate ways to give it to them. It is also our job to provide them with a lifestyle that offers them frequent opportunities to receive sensory input, explore their environment with their senses, run, jump, climb, touch, get their hands dirty, spin, etc. It is our job to let them learn through play!

> It is our job to let them LEARN THROUGH PLAY!

I want you to understand that when your children display some problems at the top of the building blocks of learning (in motor skills or performance or emotional or behavioral regulation), it doesn't mean they necessarily have a "problem"... they may simply have an immature sensory system. They just don't quite have the foundation they need and are working with a faulty structure. They need to fortify or strengthen their foundation. When they do this through enhanced opportunities for sensory input, we will often see improvements in the top of the building blocks.

Whether your child is "typically developing" has SPD, ADD/ADHD, developmental delays, is on the autism spectrum, or just has an immature sensory system, work on that sensory foundation. Build it by offering them sensory experiences throughout their day and by understanding what they need and giving them opportunities to get it. What I hope you will understand, as well, is that it is not hard. It does not cost a lot of money and does not take a lot of time. You can enhance your children's day with sensory experiences with simple, cheap, and easy strategies, tools, and techniques. It's just about making it a way of thinking and a part of your lifestyle. Once you understand it, this is all fun, easy, and best of all, a great opportunity for you to better your relationship with your child.

CONCLUSION

I want to end by telling you about one family with whom I worked and about how these strategies changed their lives. This is a story about an eight-year-old boy named Billy and a mom who "got it." Billy demonstrated some behaviors consistent with an immature sensory system and some sensory over and under-sensitivities. Homework was a struggle and often caused tears and fights. Focusing in school was a struggle. Behaviors were worrisome. I worked with Billy and his parents on ways to enhance his day with opportunities for sensory input based on what he was showing us he needed. His mom was a star pupil. She set up "stations" in their house with different sensory tools he needed and enjoyed. She used the strategies we talked about at homework time. She remembered in church or social situations that called for quiet and calm to give deep pressure or have a bag of tricks for sensory stimulation. If I said it, she did it! About a month or two into our work together, she came to me full of happy tears. She told me that they were getting through homework for the first time ever without crying and fighting. She was so excited because she felt using these strategies had improved her relationship with her son because there was less stress and conflict. She told me it actually improved her relationship with her husband and their family as a whole because they were now empowered to handle situations as they came up, to understand what was going on behind his behaviors, and to get through situations that used to be stressful but not anymore because they had the tools to handle them.

I live it every day as a mom with two kids who crave sensory input, and I see it as a clinician working with kids just like yours. I want you to be empowered to handle the challenges your children present you with and the challenges that they face and know that you have the tools to help them. Good luck and let me know how it goes!

APPENDIX A

Sensory Checklist

(Adapted from www.sensory-processing-disorder.com/sensory-processing-disorder-checklist.html)

Tactile Sense

Tactile sense: This system is our sense of touch which is gathered through our skin. It is our largest sensory system and plays an important role in behavior. There are two subsystems: the protective system and the discriminatory system. The protective system makes us scream and swat at a bug that we feel crawling on our legs or panic and pull our hand away quickly when we realize we have touched something that is hot. The discriminatory system tells us if something is hot or cold, soft or hard, bumpy or smooth, painful or pleasant, etc.

Over-sensitive to tactile input

- Seems to be fearful of or dislikes crowds
- Dislikes standing in lines or other situations where they will be in close proximity to others and risk being touched by them
- Dislikes having hair brushed
- Seems to get upset by minor injuries (cuts, bruises) or shots at the doctor's office and response is out of proportion to the severity of the stimuli
- Distressed by raindrops, water falling from the shower, running through a fountain, or other situations where water may touch their skin
- Resists touch or affection from others
- Avoids getting hands dirty or messy play (dislikes finger paint, playing in sand or mud, play-do, glue, etc.)
- Does not like to wear certain clothes (including undergarments and socks)
- Dislikes having face washed
- Distressed by having hair or nails cut
- Distressed by brushing teeth or going to the dentist

- Picky eater (avoids certain food textures)
- Walks on tiptoes
- Refuses to go barefoot in grass or sand

Under-sensitive to tactile input
- Touches everything
- Seems unaware of cuts, bumps, or bruises; has a high tolerance for pain
- Frequently bumps or pushes other children
- Bangs head, bites self, or picks nails
- Craves salty, spicy, or sour foods
- Seeks out messy play and getting their hands dirty
- Frequently puts non-food objects in their mouth
- Repeatedly touches objects or textures that they might find soothing (i.e. a favorite blanket or stuffed animal)

Difficulty with tactile discrimination and perception

Tactile discrimination: Distinguishing between the characteristics of the sensory input (hot/cold, sharp/dull, smooth/rough, etc.) Discrimination problems can lead to difficulty with skills and coordination.

Perception: Recognizing and interpreting tactile input (touch) in a way that will help us understand and learn from that input and then motivate us toward a certain action or reaction. We must correctly perceive the input to be able to make meaning out of it and apply it toward motor skills.
- Has difficulty with fine motor tasks such as buttoning, zipping, tying shoes
- Has difficulty using scissors, crayons, and silverware
- Puts things in their mouth to explore them (after the age of 2)
- Has difficulty identifying an object simply by feeling it (needs to use vision to help)

Vestibular Sense

Vestibular sense: Through information gathered via a mechanism in the inner ear, this sense tells us where our head is in relation to gravity by processing motion or change of head position. This system detects motion and gravity, and gives us our sense of balance. It can also give us information regarding the acceleration or deceleration of our bodies. This system is how we develop and comprehend the relationship of our body to the rest of the world.

Over-sensitive to vestibular input

- Prefers sedentary tasks or tasks that don't involve much physical movement
- Moves slowly and with caution
- Appears weak
- Fearful of their feet leaving the ground and of falling (even when there is no real risk involved)
- Avoids playground equipment such as swings, slides, or ladders
- Appears clumsy
- Loses balance easily
- Difficulty balancing on one foot or walking on a balance beam, curb, etc
- Avoids activities that involve spinning (i.e. merry-go-rounds, ring around the rosy, carnival rides)
- Did not like "tummy-time" as an infant
- Fearful of, or has difficulty with activities that require balance such as riding a bike or scooter
- Dislikes elevators or escalators
- Is fearful of going up or down stairs
- Gets car sick easily or frequently

Under-sensitive to vestibular input

- Always "on the go"; can't sit still
- Appears to be a "thrill-seeker"; seems to gravitate toward activities that seem dangerous
- Even while sitting, is rocking, tapping a foot, and moving around in chair
- Seeks out activities that involve movement (especially fast and intense movement)
- Could swing for days if you let them
- Does not appear to get dizzy even after long and intense episodes of spinning
- Never walks; is always running or jumping to get where they need to go
- Always jumping, spinning, or hanging upside down
- Bangs head on purpose

SENSORY CHECKLIST

Poor muscle tone or coordination

Muscle tone: Amount of tension in the muscles (not, strength, but tension)

Coordination: Gross motor or fine motor. Poor awareness of how your body is moving, will lead to coordination deficits

- Appears "floppy"; arms and legs appear hyper-flexible
- Fatigues easily
- Slumps in chair, lies head on desk, or props head on hand while seated
- "W sits"-while seated on floor vs. sitting "criss-cross applesauce"
- Has difficulty holding "superman" position (lying on stomach and simultaneously holding head up, arms up and straight out in front of them, and legs up off of the ground with straight knees)
- Has trouble catching themselves when falling
- Has difficulty putting clothes on and with buttons, zippers, tying shoes, etc.
- Bumps into things, knocks things over, or trips frequently
- Seems to have difficulty learning how to move their body to learn a new exercise, sports skill, jump over something, etc.
- Has difficulty with or is fearful of catching balls
- Has difficulty with gross motor skills such as kicking a ball, jumping jacks, hopping on one foot, etc.
- Has difficulty with fine motor skills and using "tools" such as a pencil or crayon for writing or coloring, using scissors to cut, lacing or tying shoes, using silverware to eat, etc.
- Did not crawl as an infant
- Has not established hand dominance by the age of 4 or 5

Proprioceptive Sense

Proprioceptive sense: This is our "position" sense as it processes the information gathered through our muscles, ligaments, and joints to tell us the position of our body. Proprioception helps us to motor plan (figure out what our body needs to do in order to move a certain way), have motor control (our body doing what our brain tells it to do), have postural stability and a sense of safety during movement, and allows us to grade our movements or make adjustments to the pressure, strength, or intensity we use when handling an object.

Under-sensitive to proprioceptive input/Proprioceptive seeking behaviors
- Seeks out activities that involve jumping, bumping, and crashing
- Falls on the ground purposely and frequently
- Frequently bumps, hits, or pushes others
- Chews on non-food items frequently; "shirt chewer"
- Stomps feet when walking
- Has difficulty sitting still in a chair; constantly tapping foot on floor, tapping pen on desk, etc.
- Enjoys being hugged tightly and firmly
- Loves jumping off of furniture and high places
- Loves pushing, pulling, or carrying heavy objects (such as carrying a heavy backpack, pushing a vacuum, pushing heavy furniture, pulling a wagon, etc.)
- Grinds teeth
- Would jump for hours if able
- Loves roughhousing, tackling, or wrestling
- Likes clothing to be tight

Difficulty grading movements

Grading movements: Involves making adjustments to the pressure, force, strength, or intensity needed to complete a task.
- Presses too hard when writing or erasing
- Written work is often messy
- Plays with others with too much force, often hurting them
- Seems to do everything with too much force (such as walking, slamming doors, slamming down objects, squeezing too tightly, etc.)
- Frequently breaks or drops things
- Does not seem to understand the concepts of "light" and "heavy"

Auditory Sense

Auditory sense: This system involves the information gathered through our ears. Processing of auditory information includes the ability to separate sounds heard in one ear from the other and allows us to discern sounds (such as the teacher talking from background noise in the classroom).

SENSORY CHECKLIST

Over-sensitive to auditory input
- Seems overly sensitive to sounds
- Distracted by environmental sounds (such as lawnmowers, music, people talking, etc.)
- Distracted by background noises (such as the air conditioner, a fan, a clock ticking, etc.)
- Distressed by loud noises (buzzers at a ball game, movie theater, music concerts, etc.)
- Fearful of sounds such as a hairdryer, vacuum, toilet flushing, hand dryer, dog barking, etc.
- May run away, cry, or cover ears with loud or unexpected noises

Under-sensitive to auditory input
- Does not respond to name being called
- Always making noises, talking to themselves, or humming just for the sake of making noises
- Loves loud sounds (TV, movie theaters)
- Appears oblivious to certain sounds
- Has trouble following verbal instructions

Taste And Smell
Over-sensitive to tastes and smells
- Gags with foods of certain textures
- Avoids certain tastes or smells; prefers bland food
- Resists having dental work done
- Will only eat hot or cold food
- Reacts negatively to odors in public (restaurants, stores) or at home (cooking, cleaning supplies)
- Is bothered by the scent of lotions, soaps, perfumes, and shampoos

Under-sensitive to tastes and smells
- Does not seem to notice odors and smells (which may be a safety concern)
- Prefers foods with intense flavors
- May lick, taste, or chew on inedible objects
- Does not notice unpleasant odors

Visual System
Over-sensitive to visual input
- Prefers dim lights
- Avoids eye contact
- Is distracted by other visual stimuli in the room (decorations, movement windows, etc.)
- Has difficulty keeping eyes focused on a task for an appropriate amount of time

Under-sensitive to visual input
- Has difficulty following a moving object, such as a ball, with their eyes
- May complain of having tired eyes
- Often loses their place while reading or copying written work
- Has difficulty locating objects among other items (clothes in a drawer, food on a shelf, toys in a bin, etc.)
- Reverses certain words or letters when copying or reads words backwards after the first grade (such as "on" for "no" or "top" for "pot")

Interoceptive System

Interoceptive sense: This system provides us with sensations from internal sensors near our organs including our heart, stomach, bowel, and bladder. It tells us how we feel inside as it gives us information regarding our heart rate, hunger, thirst, digestion, state of arousal, mood, etc.

- Has frequent muscle aches or pain
- Frequently complaining of vague discomfort
- Severe mood swings with moods that can change quickly
- Difficulty regulating thirst or hunger; always thirsty/hungry or never thirsty/hungry
- Difficulty potty training; does not seem to feel the sensation when it is time to go
- Can switch quickly from one state of arousal to another (i.e. lethargic to hyper, overstimulated to under stimulated)

Self-Regulation

Self-regulation: Self-regulation is the way in which we manage and cope with situations that are emotional in nature; situations that require us to monitor, adapt to, or change how we act or react on a moment to moment basis.

- Difficulty getting along with peers
- Prefers playing alone
- Difficulty accepting changes in routine
- Easily frustrated
- Impulsive
- Uses tantrums to express themselves
- Avoids eye contact
- Has difficulty playing independently (needs adult guidance) over the age of 18 months
- Excessive irritability or fussiness as an infant
- Has difficulty self-soothing/calming
- Has difficulty falling asleep; needs a lot of adult help to calm self in order to go to sleep
- Wakes up frequently through the night and needs adult help to go back to sleep
- Has difficulty forming bonds/relationships with familiar people

BIBLIOGRAPHY

Ayres, A.J. (1979). Sensory Integration and the Child. Los Angeles, CA: Northwestern Psychological Services.

Bailer, D.S., Miller, L.J. (2011). No Longer A Secret: Unique Common Sense Strategies for Children with Sensory and Motor Challenges. Sensory World: Arlington Texas.

Baker, A. E., Lane A., Angley M. T., Young R. L. (2008). The relationship between sensory processing patterns and behavioural responsiveness in autistic disorder: a pilot study. Journal of Autism and Developmental Disorders, 38, 867–875. doi: 10.1007/s10803-007-0459-0.

Baranek G. T., David F. J., Poe M. D., Stone W. L., Watson L. R. (2006). Sensory experiences questionnaire: discriminating sensory features in young children with autism, developmental delays, and typical development. Journal of Child Psychology and Psychiatry, 47, 591–601. doi: 10.1111/j.1469-7610.2005.01546.x.

Ben-Sasson, A, Briggs-Gowan, M.J., Carter, A.S. (2009). Sensory Over-Responsivity in Elementary Schools: Prevalence and Social Emotional Correlates. Journal of Abnormal Child Psychology, 37:705-716. doi: 10.1007/s 10802-008-9295-8.

Bundy, A.C., Lane, S.J., Murray, E.A. (2002). Sensory Integration: Theory and Practice, (2nd 3d). F.A. Davis Company: Philadelphia, PA.

Chapman, J. (2009). Sensory Processing Disorder and Children with Autism: Understanding the problem. Retrieved January 20, 2013 from: http://voices.yahoo.com/sensory-processing-disorder-children-autism-3158451.html?cat=70.

Gopnik, A., Meltzoff, A. N., Kuhl, P. K. (1999). The Scientist in the Crib: Minds, Brains, and

How Children Learn. New York, NY: William Morrow and Company, Inc.

Jensen, E. (2005). Teaching with the Brain in Mind (2nd edition). Associations for Supervision and Curriculum Development: Alexandria, VA.

Kranowitz, C.S. (2006) The Out of Sync Child. New York, NY: Berkley Publishing Group.

Leekam S. R., Libby S. J., Wing L., Gould J. (2007). Describing the sensory abnormalities of children and adults with autism. Journal of Autism and Developmental Disorders, 37, 894–910. doi: 10.1007/s10803-006-0218-7.

Minsky, M. (1986). The Society of the Mind. Simon and Schuster Inc; New York, NY.

Obesity in children and teens. American Academy of Child and Adolescent Psychiatry, No. 79 (2011). Retrieved May, 2013 from www.aacap.org.

Oden. A. (2006) Ready Bodies Learning Minds 2nd Edition. Spring Branch, TX: David Oden.

Rosemond, J. Ritalin isn't only cure for child. Article in the Albuquerque Journal Newspaper, June 4, 1998.

Shore, S.M. (2004). Focus on...autism: Perception. S.I. Focus, Summer, 2004, 17-20.

Shore, S.M., Grandin, T. (2003). Beyond the Wall: Personal Experiences with Autism and Asperger Syndrome (2nd edition). Autism Asperger Publishing Co: Shawnee Mission, KS.

Sicile-Kira, C. (2008). Autism Life Skills: From Communication and Safety to Self-Esteem and More-10 Essential Abilities Every Child Needs and Deserves to Learn. Penguin Group: New York, New York.

Stockman, I. (2004). Movement and Action in Learning Development: Clinical Implications for Pervasive Developmental Disorders: Elseveir Academic Press: San Diego, CA.

BIBLIOGRAPHY

Talay-Ongan, A, and Wood, K. (2000). Unusual sensory sensitivities in autism: a possible crossroads. International Journal of Disability Development and Education. 47(2), 201-202.

Temple University Health Sciences Center (2005, May 13). Study Finds ADHD Improves with Sensory Intervention. Science Daily. Retrieved September 4, 2013 from www.sciencedaily.com/releases/2005/05/050513103548.htm

Tomchek S. D., Dunn W. (2007). Sensory processing in children with and without autism: a comparative study using the short sensory profile. American Journal of Occupational Therapy. 61, 190–200.

Trott, M.C., Laurel, M,K., Windeck, S.L. (1993) SenseAbilities: Understanding Sensory Integration. San Antonio, TX: Therapy Skill Builders.

VanSant, A. Concepts of Neural Organization and Movement. In: Connolly, B., Montgomery, P. Therapeutic Exercises in Developmental Disabilities. 3rd ed. Thorofare, NJ. SLACK Inc; 2005:1-20

Made in the USA
Columbia, SC
29 November 2019

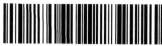